Praise for David Bernstein, MD

I've Got Some Good News and Some Bad News: YOU'RE OLD...

A geriatrician's lively guide to living well after 60.

Bernstein loves counseling and treating the elderly. He's fascinated by "how we live our lives and what we do near the end that makes [life] significant." Here, he shares—through his experiences with patients and family—his enthusiasm and respect for the process of aging. His guiding philosophy is to keep the ultimate end in mind as he helps the aged cope, in a sensible, realistic way, with the multiple, difficult issues of old age. For a healthy, fulfilling life, he encourages the understanding and practice of what he calls the five attributes of GRACE: Goals, Roots (as in DNA), Attitude, Companionship and Environment (as in lifestyle). Throughout the chapters, Bernstein shares anecdotes of elders working into old age, living to be 100, having sex after 70, and driving (or not) at 80 and up. The guide touches on a range of topics facing the geriatric population: cancer, heart disease, dementia, changes in living arrangements, hospice care, doctor–patient relationships and loss of independence. Each chapter ends with notes for living longer and more gracefully, as well as a list of resources and links for further exploration. In a caring but unsentimental manner, the guide makes it clear that, indeed, there's no way out of this business of aging and reaching the end of life. Bernstein has come to realize that "[o]lder adults are desperate to be heard and understood," so he has listened without judgment, asked questions, learned about his patients and figured out "how to live a long and fulfilling life." A necessary, fresh, straightforward read for all ages, since life, as Bernstein bluntly states, is a process of coming-of-old-age.

KIRKUS BOOK REVIEW

D1566550

"In my estimation, Dr. Bernstein successfully achieved his goal to express useful ideas that may help us age GRACEfully. His five themes, conditions, patient types, and philosophies established Bernstein's creative style but more than that demonstrated the depth of thought from Bernstein. This indeed led me to look at what other gems might be hidden within his manuscript. My discovery left me without disappointment. Bernstein has shared with us his growth at becoming a physician with the capacity to be both empathetic and constructively objective while working with his patients. What speaks volumes is Dr. Bernstein's ability to actively listen and communicate with his patients. This skill is not easy to master and the gift of shared expression is one that all professions will find beneficial."

Mary Dee Snow, Ph.D, MA, LMT. age 58 Clearwater, Florida

" How good it is to know that life, when we are older, can be more than just going to doctors to stay alive, and how wonderful it is to know that there are doctors whose wisdom and devotion can do more than keep us alive, more than keep us functioning. There are doctors who help us find new meaning and new joy in life, no matter our age."

Rabbi Gary Klein, age 62 Temple Ahavat Shalom, Palm Harbor, Florida

"As one who is entering my 60s, Dr. Bernstein's GRACE is an easy to remember acronym for how I want to age. In life, I find the best lessons are watching others and Dr. Bernstein's stories of his patients provided a wonderful education and much for me to think about in the years ahead. This book also helped me think about my parents and the conversations I will be having in the years ahead."

Jane Aronoff, age 59 Marietta, Georgia

"This is a delightful book that is hard to put down. Dr. Bernstein is a gifted writer whose stories of his patients reflects not only his compassion and concern for his patients but also the love that sustains many elderly couples through the illnesses and challenges they face. Bernstein weaves together stories from his own family life with those of his patients. The result is a book that is both engaging and life-affirming."

Roy Sandstrom, age 75 Clearwater, Florida

"Probably, because I always dreamed that medicine should be practiced as you described it in your book " I've Got Some Good News and Some Bad News YOU'RE OLD", I found it to be very exciting and stimulating. Chapter 8, Beginning with the End in Mind was especially thought provoking as I had avoided family conferences involving terminal care as I felt defeated in my fight to win the contest between life and death. I see that I short changed my patients and wish that could do it over. However, I am happy to see that a strong advocate of increased compassion such as yours is active and will improve the quality of our medical practicing."

Alan Goldfarb, MD age 87 Retired Physician, Buffalo, New York

"Dr. Bernstein's long tenure in the field of geriatric medicine has provided him with a wealth of knowledge in managing care for our senior citizens. His gentle approach to the issue of senior driving privileges provided me with a measure of comfort when it came time to manage my own mother's driving issues. He is truly a resource in the field of geriatrics."

Robert Bandes, age 65 Oldsmar, Florida

"Your book is a Gold Mind for an older person intent of making progress in their daily life… A work of art by a master in the medical profession…."

Reg Laskey, age 88 Detroit, MI

"Your book will be an inspiration to me to age gracefully. I shall keep on "Dancing as Fast as I can" and remember that it is not just getting old, it is "Aging GRACEfully"."

V. Smith, age 87 Clearwater Florida

"…I found your book spoke to me personally because I so admire and care for our elderly and their circumstances in growing old. You respectfully share true life as it is presented to you….As you pointed out; you have to employ humility in guiding those before you."

Clare Bennett, age 49 Owner, South Tampa Elder Support

"Educational and Inspiring…a philosophical look into the enduring understandings one physician enjoys from knowing and treating his aging patients. In his professional, yet humorous expertise, Dr. Bernstein shares this valuable knowledge with his readers, which translates into meaningful suggestions for a happy, healthy longevity."

Rosemary Lenahan age 66, Palm Harbor, Florida

"This was wonderful book and I thoroughly enjoyed it. It flowed smoothly, read easily, and wove a wonderful fabric of useful information -- much of which I already knew from having worked in social services for 35 years but was glad to have reinforced -- and some learning that I know will be useful in the years ahead. There were parts of the book that were personal for me -- like the time I had to take the car keys from my father because his macular degeneration posed a threat to others. The book provides valuable insights and about the many issues of contemporary aging. This is a book for those with aging parents, and everyone else as they age."

Harvey Landress age 62, Seminole, Florida

"… I read and experienced exactly what the title "prepared" me for… what to expect in the years to come. Aging is not something to fear - and the practical, emotional and GRACEfull advice (and anecdotal stories) were wonderfully entertaining and full of important information at the same time."

Cindy Dryce age, 50 Palm Harbor, Florida

"Each of the experiences you describe with a patient is solved with the skill, patience, and understanding that my family and I have come to know at your hands for over ten years…Although it is probably necessary for our medical advisor to distance his personal life from patients' curiosity, it was still very interesting to read about your sons, and your siblings and your parents. .....the book is also a helpful resource, with the lists at the end of each chapter."

M. Gianacakes, age 80 Clearwater, Florida

".....at the end I had a positive feeling about getting old and dying gracefully… It was also very clear that you enjoy the work you do, the interactions you have with most of your patients, and that you are dedicated to treating them with compassion, dignity and with a goal to help them "live" a productive and dignified life, even in their dying days.

Michael Rehr, Esq., age 58 Miami, Florida

I've Got Some Good News and Some Bad News:

YOU'RE OLD

OLD

TALES OF A GERIATRICIAN
WHAT TO EXPECT IN
YOUR 60s, 70s, 80s,
AND BEYOND

DAVID BERNSTEIN, M.D.

Published in the United States by Dynamic Learning

Paperback ISBN-13: 978-0-9907087-0-4
eBook ISBN-13: 978-0-9907087-1-1

Books are available in quantity for promotional or premium branded corporate use.

For more information on discounts, terms and media requests contact:

Dynamic Learning
Media Department
314 Shore Dr. E. Oldsmar, Florida 34677-3916
Melissa@davidbernsteinmd.com

Visit us at www.davidbernsteinmd.com

Author's Note

In order to protect the privacy of those mentioned in this book, names and certain identifying characteristics of most patients whose medical histories are described have been changed. Furthermore all stories were written following HIPAA (Health Portability Act of 1996) compliance guidelines.

Table of Contents

Introduction

Why I Practice Geriatric Medicine

Age is not a particularly interesting subject. Anyone can get old. All you have to do is live long enough.
– Groucho Marx

You know you're getting old when all the names in your black book have M.D. after them.
– Arnold Palmer

You can't help getting older, but you don't have to get old.
– George Burns

I am frequently asked what attracts me to taking care of the elderly. The answer is neither simple nor the same everyday. It certainly is not for the money. A long time ago the great philosopher, "my mother," told me to become a dermatologist. If she was referring to money and life style, she was right. The only problem is that it did not meet my needs: It did not satisfy my inquisitive nature or my constant need for challenge nor did it satisfy my need to connect with people and learn

1

from them. Through my work I have had the wonderful opportunity to hear about my patients' successes and failures, their ups and their downs. Over the years, they have confided in me about deeply personal events—an experience during WWII; a new intimate relationship at the age of 80; the sadness of placing a spouse in a nursing home. What had worked in their personal and professional lives? What was working for them in their retirement? Best of all, I find that I am able to pass these valuable lessons on to others in my practice.

One of these experiences happened after I had been in practice for about 10 years. But before I get into the story, I must admit that I have been a baseball fan all my life. My friend Jim is even more of a fan than I am. Together we have had the good fortune to live out a dream.

When spring training begins in Florida, many of the teams need physicians to perform physicals on the major league and minor league players. As a result of Jim's persistence and connections, he and I have had this opportunity. Not only is it a thrill for me to have seen some of my idols who are now coaches and managers, and the young and talented players of today's era; I also got to see my friend Jim become a little kid while he was doing this job.

Once, when we were in Lakeland doing this "job" for the Detroit Tigers, I watched Jim become awestruck at the sight of Al Kaline, his boyhood idol. This was followed by a rectal exam performed on Al Kaline, the "patient." That same morning Jim walked up to the manager of the Detroit Tigers, Sparky Anderson, and asked for an autograph. I have never forgotten the moment when Jim said, "Mr. Anderson, may I please have your autograph?" Sparky, a white-haired gentleman wearing his baseball uniform, responded, "My father is 'Mr. Anderson'; I'm Sparky. Sure Doc, I'd be happy to."

Performing these physicals has become a Spring ritual for Jim and me and we both find that it is one of the highlights of our year. In recent years we have limited our work to the Toronto Blue Jays as their spring training complex is very close to our offices. I look forward to the phone call I get from Jim every year telling me what day and time we will be doing our "job."

One year was particularly interesting; in addition to working for the Toronto Blue Jays we were asked to perform exams on the *World Champion* New York Yankees minor league players. How could I refuse? I grew up in New York and the Yankees had won the World Series just a few months earlier. The process is very much like an assembly line, especially when doing this for the minor league players. They go through a dental exam, X-rays, eye exam, TB skin test, EKG, and blood testing before I even see a player. After I have completed my portion of the exam, they see an orthopedist and who knows what after that. On that morning, from 7:00 a.m. to noon, I examined **75** twenty - year old young men. Most had the same life experiences. They loved baseball, played it from the time they could walk, and were playing in the minor leagues with the hope that one day they would make it "to the show." By the time the morning was over, I had had a great time and gotten paid for having fun but I left without making any real connections with any of these men.

I rushed back to my office with little time to spare, and I skipped lunch as my afternoon schedule was packed; I had twenty **75**-year old patients. I found the morning thrilling for what is was—a chance to mingle with potential future superstars, but I found the afternoon, which was full of older adults with chronic medical problems, far more stimulating. They had stories that were twice as old as the young boys I had seen in the morning and there was meaning to their lives.

Carson was my last patient of the day. Most of the time he wanted to be seen early in the day or he called to be seen urgently. He had been feeling tired recently. I had adjusted some medication three weeks earlier to see if his symptoms would respond to drugs for congestive heart failure. I was really uncertain. The choice of medicine—Coreg—was a diagnostic challenge as much as anything else.

Carson, a widower, had been a patient for many years and very appreciative of the care I'd given him and his wife before she died. I had gained Carson's confidence early as he had confided in me that he gets very severe anxiety attacks. After observing these severe episodes I began to see a pattern. They frequently occurred after some type of tragic news was reported by the news media. As I gained insight, Carson told me that he was a survivor of the Bataan death march. I nodded my head; I was embarrassed that I did not know what that was but it certainly did not sound like it had been an enjoyable experience. (I went home that night and read all that I could find about it to be better prepared for our next encounter). Carson had become a prisoner of war while serving in the Philippines during WWII. During his imprisonment he was tortured and his weight dropped to below 100 pounds. He told me that he does not like to speak about those events and shares this information with no one. When I suggested that he visit the VA clinic as they have a specialist who could help him, he told me that it makes him much worse to relive the past. He confided in me when episodes trigger these panic attacks and requested some medication to control them. The panic attacks were becoming more frequent as world events were vividly described on TV 24-hours a day. Thank goodness I found a medication that worked most of the time. Carson has been leading a more peaceful existence. Even into his 80s, and despite several cardiac stents, he is able to travel and visit family across the country.

Now Carson is in my office late in the day, my last patient. I had been up since 5:00 a.m. I had made my hospital rounds before working at the Yankee complex and I was tired but I had enough strength for Carson. He tells me that he is feeling better but adds, "Doc, I don't think it has anything to do with the new medicine Coreg because I only took it for a few days." I tried to keep a poker face and not show my disappointment or that I was puzzled. I noticed that Carson's lips had separated a bit and he had a content look on his face. Then I said, "So Carson, if it is not the medicine, why is it that you feel so much better?" A different smile appeared on his face as he told me that he had met a woman a few weeks ago, a widow. They had gone to lunch and dinner a few times and he was enjoying her company. They had some things in common including family back in Michigan. His smile got bigger as he told me that last night she invited him back to her "double wide" and said, "Carson, my husband had been ill for several years before he died. I have not had sex in 16 years. Would you like to sleep with me tonight?"

I don't get surprised very often but my chin dropped. I am very used to this subject matter; I enjoy speaking to my patients about sex; but the way she presented her desire was unique. Carson then saw a big grin on my face, matching his. I asked if there was anything else I could do as it seemed like things were going very well for him. He replied, "Yes doc. She is going to her doctor today to make some inquiries about how it can be more pleasurable for her. How about some Viagra for me?"

This was a day I will always cherish, and it stands as one of the reasons I love my job.

It is questions like these that individuals struggle with every day as they age.

What happens as we age—physically, mentally, and socially? What are the abilities of medicine and its limits? What are the social issues adults face as they become elderly? All of these are the issues I grapple with each day and it is endlessly fascinating.

Life is an aging process. Each of us goes through it in different ways, and it is how we live our lives and what we do near the end that makes it significant. In this way, my patients unknowingly serve as guides for me. They share with me the good, the bad, and the ugly. When we can, we find humor in the challenges. When we can't, caring and respect carry us along together to an unexpected place of enlightenment.

Notes on living longer:

- As we mature and gain experiences we have a chance to grow, mature and enjoy life.
- Smell the roses and the garbage—incorporate life experiences into your being.

- If we are lucky we can experience our dreams or joyful events that we can cherish while painful and unfortunate events will shape our lives as well.
- Put experiences to good use. Learn to celebrate when your dreams come true and don't be afraid to reach for what you want in life. You might live to regret lost opportunitiesWe grow by learning to overcome painful experiences and by incorporating joyful ones.

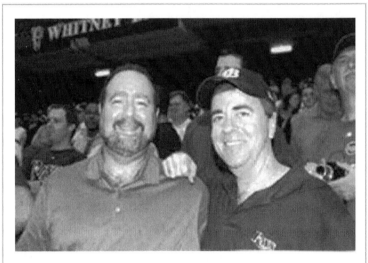

THE AUTHOR AND FRIEND JIM AT
BASEBALL GAME TOGETHER

Chapter 1

GRACE is a 5 Letter Word
Living it up to live longer

Old age isn't so bad when you consider the alternative.
– Maurice Chevalier

Growing old is mandatory; growing up is optional.
– Chili Davis

Through my early adulthood, the number 5 had no particular significance in my life; however, as a young boy growing up, a favorite number revolved around famous athletes. Forty-one was my favorite number because the all-star pitcher for the New York Mets, Tom Seaver, proudly wore that number. When I had a chance to choose a uniform number as a high school athlete, I chose the number 24 because that was the number Willie Mays and Bill Bradley wore (number 41 was too high and was rarely available). If the number 24 was not available I took number 12, which was half of 24. In reality, the number was really no big deal; I was just happy to make the team.

What is it about the number 5, then? As I thought about it, my immediate family had 5 members: mother, father, sister, brother, and me. As a youth, I gravitated to a sport comprised of 5 players: basketball. Probably the most important association has to do with the five fingers on my hand. I am really "attached" to them and I find they are an easy number to count off whatever I'm trying to remember or categorize.

During my medical residency, I had the opportunity to learn from many brilliant scholars. One of these mentors gave me this advice: "When you complete a consultation on a patient, limit your recommendations to five. It is just too difficult for the doctor reading the consultation to follow more than 5 recommendations at one time. If you wish, come back tomorrow with 5 more recommendations."

Curiously, as I delved into books about health and fitness, I continually again came across the number 5. In the book *5 Factor Fitness* personal trainer Harly Pasternak put together an exercise system that revolved around the number 5. Five themes or philosophies were incorporated into many of his teachings, such as 5 sets of exercise—each lasting 5 minutes, 5 days a week. He also recommends 5 small meals a day, each one containing 5 ingredients. In his book *Body Rx*, A. Scott Connelly instructs the reader to list 6 favorite foods or meals, suggesting that as we go through life getting fat, we eat the same 6 foods all the time. I performed the exercise and was stumped. As much as I like to eat, I could not make a list of more than 5 items in any given category that I routinely ate.

What about other groupings of 5, I wondered? My life's "jobs": family member, friend, student, teacher, and doctor. Exercises I perform: strength training, cardio, individual sport (golf), group sport (basketball), eastern techniques (Yoga, Tai Chi, meditation). I just love lists of 5s, and I can almost always remember 5 things.

In the short vignettes later in this chapter and the longer stories in the chapters that follow, I detail the lives of patients who demonstrate the 5 attributes that I have observed which lead to longer, happier lives. The reader will also find throughout the chapters the concepts of five as a recurring theme: 5 *basic patient types*, 5 *philosophies*, 5 *major diseases*, and 5 *themes* running though most of the stories.

5 THEMES

1. Patients are human—full of the same emotions we all experience every day.
2. Making important decisions is difficult and complicated.
3. A sense of fulfillment in life is essential.
4. As humans, we all have a need to be heard and acknowledged.
5. We need connections to others.

After years of practice as a geriatrician, I noticed that I was treating 5 different conditions every day.

5 CONDITIONS

1. Metabolic and vascular disorders such as diabetes, high cholesterol, hypertension and heart ailments.
2. Bone disorders such as osteoporosis, arthritis, spinal stenosis.
3. Psychological disorders such as depression, anxiety, family dynamics and emotional problems.
4. Geriatric disorders such as problems with memory, falls, urinating, loss of independence, grief, and end of life.
5. Health maintenance such as disease prevention testing, counseling on obesity, smoking, diet, exercise and accident prevention.

Furthermore, I have reflected on the 5 different types of patients I see day in and day out.

5 PATIENT TYPES

1. The angry, negative pessimist: the patient who feels that whatever happens to him is someone else's fault.
2. The inattentive, non-adherent: the patient who takes advice from other, less informed, individuals but not his/her physician.
3. The analytical engineer types: constantly questioning my rationale.
4. The compliant: "Yes, doctor, whatever you say".
5. The argumentative patient.

I also want to share with you 5 philosophies that I consistently use in my approach to people, and in patient care. They are part of my overall approach in life and are really quite simple.

5 PHILOSOPHIES

1. "Common things *are* common." I learned this from my chief resident as an intern. It became ingrained as it was repeated almost every day during our "morning report" for three years. There is a longer version and one that has you visualize yourself in a field with the sound of hoof beats and you ask yourself if the sound is that of a horse or a zebra. Since horses are more likely to be present, the exercise has you concentrate on the more common phenomena to occur.
2. "Begin with the end in mind." This is an approach I learned from Dr. Stephen Covey in one of his many books. It teaches you to look at the final result you are aiming for and work backward to develop a solution.

3. "As we get older we become more of what we were."
   I learned this from the great philosopher in my life,
   Mom. She believes that as people age the only way in
   which they change is to become a more exaggerated
   version of themselves.

4. "A test is only as good as the question you are asking."
   This is another pearl of wisdom I learned during
   my internship and residency; it regards the fact that
   one has to carefully think before ordering any test as
   to what the outcome will be and how it will help or
   hinder the evaluation of the patient. In other words,
   don't order a test if you don't know what to do with the
   result when it comes in.

5. "If you ask enough questions and listen carefully,
   your patient will tell you what is wrong." This is self-
   explanatory: it means that if you have patience in your
   interaction with your patients and allow them to speak
   with as few interruptions as possible, they will provide
   enough information to make a diagnosis 95 percent of
   the time even without an exam or a single test.

The preceding grouping of fives has evolved over my many
years in practice, although many were inspired during my medical
education and training. I arrived at my next listing—those attributes
of my patients who have lived happy and long lives—when I was
asked by Judy Stump, the community relations coordinator of a local
retirement community, to give a workshop for her residents and the
local community. Since it was an invitation without a specific topic, I
was on my own. When she described how active the residents in her
community were, I decided to call my address "Living it up to live
longer: secrets I have learned about longevity." As I prepared for my
presentation, I thought it would be helpful to use an acronym to hold

the attention of the octogenarians in the audience. I hadn't anticipated the challenge of developing an acronym for the subject that I was proposing to address. I planned an interactive session with the group and to start by asking the elder adults in attendance a few questions. I realized that this audience would have more life experience than I as they were all a minimum of 25 years older. I had questions in mind, such as what did they think "living it up to live longer" meant? Why should I be giving a workshop when they had more life experiences than I? Since living it up and living longer meant possibly living to be 100, did anyone really want to live to 100? Before I knew it, they ended up telling me what their secrets were and lo, and behold, they matched my list as well. As the program became lively, I realized how "graced" I was to be a participant with such a group and that's when I discovered my acronym: GRACE.

It just so happened, and not to my surprise, that my acronym ended up being five letters (as mentioned earlier I have been focused on the number 5 for quite some time). The following are the five attributes of GRACE I find helpful to living it up to live longer: **G**oals, **R**oots, **A**ttitude/**A**dventure, **C**ompanionship/**C**onnections, and **E**nvironment.

Goal—having a purpose in life. A goal gives an individual a direction in life, a reason to go on living, providing rewards beyond just financial.

Roots—having the right genetic make-up, heredity, DNA. I frequently remind my patients that they chose the right (or wrong) parents.

Attitude—keeping positive about life and also about being adventurous.

Companionship/Connections—love, intimacy, and bonds with family and friends enrich your life.

Environment—leading a healthy life, paying attention to fitness, being cautious, and listening to the advice of health professionals can enable you to live longer and better.

G—GOALS

As my practice matured and I got to know my patients, the subject of their retirement would come up. I would be quick to offer my advice: that they save their money, adopt hobbies, and have plans for what they would do for the rest of their lives. Having Goals or a purpose or a hobby would be essential ingredients for a happy retirement.

I recall a story my patient Robert told to me about his retirement. He had a job that was physically demanding and when he came home at the end of the day dinner was always ready. Once he was retired, he did not have a goal, hobby or purpose in life so he assumed the role of "supervisor" for his wife Alice. His long, awaited and well-deserved retirement did not get off to a good start. He was used to the role of supervisor and she thrived on her independence. Here they were, a happily married couple *until* he retired and invaded her space. With no interests other than his work and no purpose to his life, he became a miserable man looking for someone or something to supervise.

R—ROOTS

Angelo had been a patient for 10 years or so and was in his mid 80s when he made a remark one day that took me by surprise. During a routine exam, he implied that he expected to live to be 100. Even though he was in very good health I inquired why he thought he would live that long *and* if he really wanted to. To my surprise, he told me that in fact, yes, he did want to live to be 100 and he expected to because both his parents lived that long. I considered it a daunting task to help this man live another 15 years. We discussed it further. He told me that he found life to be very enjoyable—he had a wonderful family and he felt great. He reminded me that his only real medical problem was his enlarged prostate gland, mild hypertension, and gray hair. He told me that he did not see these as impediments to living to be 100. I gave it some consideration and told him I would support his effort.

Later in the day I reflected upon Angelo's desire to live to be 100 years old. What was so outlandish about that? One of the most striking observations I've made during my years in practice has been the role that genes, DNA and heredity have on illness and longevity. It's been my pleasure to observe this in both physical attributes as well as psychological and behavioral attributes. In my years as a doctor I have had the opportunity to treat parents, grandparents, and grandchildren and see just how much of a role heredity and genes play in health, wellness, and spirit.

A—ATTITUDE

Attitude, gratitude (which is an attitude) and adventure are key ingredients to living it up and living longer. My patients who live with positive attitudes often have a sense that their age or birthdate has no bearing on how they should live their lives.

One such patient was Joanne. At each visit she had a smile on her face; she looked forward to every day no matter what was dealt her. She and her husband did not have much money; she worked for a realtor friend prepping homes that were to be put up for sale. While the realtor had become very successful and made a lot of money, she had sadness in her life as she had been widowed twice. Joanne lived with her husband in a modest house but she did enjoy driving the sports car her husband had leased. She played golf and enjoyed traveling. She would often take off just to visit a friend half way across the country. She got a big smile on her face one day when she said," Doc, you won't believe it but I just spent the past 2 weeks painting a 3,000-square foot home and applying wall paper to 3 gigantic bathrooms with 10-foot ceilings." "Joanne," I asked, "what will you do next?" With a grin, she told me she was going to play golf for the next 2 weeks to "recover from that back-breaking work."

Joanne trusted me with her innermost thoughts, which mainly had to with living her life to the fullest. One day she asked if she could entrust the care of her husband to me. She warned me that he would be a bad patient in that he smoked, drank and did not listen to advice from anyone—including doctors! He was everything she told me he would be. He, too, enjoyed life very much. They were well suited to each other. Unfortunately, before I could scratch the surface of his several serious medical conditions, he died. Happily, I presume, because it occurred while he was smoking a cigarette, in his garage, with his beloved car.

Joanne went through a fairly normal grieving process and she, understandably, was angry with her deceased husband for leaving her—especially with debt, no life insurance, and a leased sports car she would have to return. She got over the anger quickly, though, stating, "That's just life, Doc. You gotta go on." Eight months after his death, she sold her home, put all her belongs in storage, packed up her car and made a visit to my office. "Doc, I'm going on a trip," she exclaimed.

"Where are you headed?" I asked.

"Well, Doc, I have friends in 13 states between here and Oregon and they have always asked me to visit them. Now is the time. I am off in 2 days." I looked at her with a mix of disbelief and envy.

"What a gutsy thing for you to do. Who are you going with?" I asked.

"Just by myself. I am a real adventurer at heart, and my friends are great. We'll have a great time wherever I go."

Some months later she did come back for a visit to my office for me to check on her blood pressure and then told me she was off again. This time to North Carolina to manage a restaurant owned by her son, as he and his wife were going to spend 6 months in Europe.

C—COMPANIONSHIP

Companionship has to do with having strong personal relationships and intimacy. I have had the great fortune to observe this dynamic among many couples I have taken care of over the years. It is that special bond that holds people together, the sharing of raising children or having a pet or working together professionally or on community projects.

Mary Brown brought her parents to my office one day after they moved them from Delaware to Florida. I had known Mary for many years as our children went to the same school, but prior to this visit I had never met her parents. They had been married for 60 years. He was a very intelligent man and had been involved in planning and engineering while living in Delaware. His wife, a very supportive woman, was his pride and joy. At their first visit, Mary told me how devoted they were to one another and how protective they were of one another as well. The reason they had moved was that they could no longer take care of themselves as they both had dementia and he had heart problems. They were a cute, adorable and endearing couple for the entire time I took care of them.

Mary and others who knew them well would describe them as inseparable. They covered up for each other's cognitive shortcomings, which ultimately made it difficult to figure out exactly what was going on in their lives. As time went on, his bathing and grooming habits deteriorated and she became very protective of his desire to remain in the same clothes all the time. She would make excuses for this behavior. One day, she fell while getting into a car to come to my office and fractured her hip. This incident was the beginning of the end for this couple who had never been separated, except when she had been in the hospital to deliver their two children. Fortunately, her hospitalization was short but she needed to be in a nursing home to recover. The husband was beside himself with loneliness. I had never truly realized just how close these two people were until I learned from administrators at their retirement community and the nursing home that they were constantly holding hands. To my disbelief, when I inquired further, I was informed that despite their older age and maladies, they slept in the same bed and held hands all night long; when they were at the dinner table, they constantly gazed into each other's eyes. What love they had for each other! Their companionship supported them and kept them independent and alive.

E—ENVIRONMENT

The environment in which we live plays a major role in how we maintain our health. The choices people make to practice healthy lifestyles are key attributes to a longer, happier and more fulfilling life. In my practice, I tend to see more people who have *unhealthy* habits because as people make poor or unhealthy choices, it leads to more illness and need for medical care. Did you know that over the past 50 years the following 5 things have grown at the same rate: the number of fast food restaurants, the number of television stations, the percentage of the population with obesity, the number of diabetics, and the number of prescriptions for antidepressants? These are alarming statistics that indicate the role of environment in health and longevity.

Betty is a 72-year-old patient whom I have treated for several years. She has been resistant to accepting my interventions to improve her health and reduce her potential to die of a heart attack. She is obese, has diabetes and high cholesterol—and she smokes. Her diet is unrestricted and she does not exercise. She pleads with me for one more chance every time I recommend placing her on more medication. She is unwilling or unable to make any lifestyle changes to reduce her risk—she simply will not change her *environment*. Yet, her environment will kill her. On the other hand, I do have countless patients who see me very infrequently as they have created favorable environments for themselves.

Robin is one of my patients who takes her health very seriously. She is a slender, 48-year-old married woman and mother of 2 teenage boys. In the 20-plus years I have known her she has been a great example of what I mean by interacting well with the environment. She has maintained her ideal body weight, performs both cardiovascular

exercises and yoga a minimum of 2 days each a week. She eats a low fat, mostly organic diet free of high-fructose products.

She has an annual exam including a mammogram and takes the opportunity to review her tests results carefully. When I diagnosed her with an underactive thyroid condition she educated herself on the condition and resisted taking medication for a few months before consenting to follow the advice of her physician (me). She makes sure to get the proper amount of sleep every night (7 to 8 hours) and she flosses her teeth daily (no doubt because she is a dental hygienist).

Within each of my stories, you will find one or more of the themes, philosophies and patient types mentioned here that I see every day in my practice. My challenge is to synthesize all the information during a patient visit and make clinical judgments while formulating a comprehensive plan with the patient. These are welcome challenges that provide me with a great sense of accomplishment and fulfillment.

Notes for living longer

- Have goals throughout your life.
- Recognize how your family medical history (your "roots") might affect your health and work with your doctor to improve and protect your health.
- Keep a positive attitude about life and also about being safely adventurous.
- Nourish your connections with friends and family so that you can experience love, intimacy, and bonds throughout life.
- Create a healthy life by paying attention to your environment; maintain fitness, be judicious in your lifestyle habits, and listen to the advice of health professionals who can help you live longer, and better!

Resources and Links:

Chopra, Deepak & Simon, David (2001) *Grow Younger, Live Longer*, New York, Three Rivers Press a division of Random House, Inc.

Helpguide.org, *Healthy Aging Tips: How to Feel Young and Live Life to the Fullest*, retrieved November 3, 2011 from www.helpguide.org/life/healthy_aging_seniors_aging_well.htm

Moseley, Lorimer (2011, Jan 3) Bodymind.org, *Keeping your Brain Active in Old Age,* Retrieved October, 2011 from http://Bodymind.org//novelty-exercise-and-diet-the-cornerstones-of-neural-and-cognitive-plasticity/

Chapter 2

Working into Old Age

How old would you be if you didn't know how old you were?
– **Satchel Paige**

To find joy in work is to discover the fountain of youth.
– **Pearl S. Buck**

I want to be all used up when I die.
– **George Bernard Shaw**

Getting through medical school and residency is a daunting task and when I completed that, I embarked on one even more difficult—starting an Internal Medicine practice. I sought out many advisors and learned there were many facets to consider. Retirement planning came up fairly early. While I recognized that what this really meant was buying all types of insurance, it did give me cause to consider that there would come a day when I would not be going to the hospital or my office. What a glorious idea; up to this point life had been 12 years of public school (filled with anxiety about making the basketball team and getting into a good college), four years of college (filled with apprehensions about getting into medical school), four years of medical school (filled with the fear of killing a patient) and then one year of internship and two years of Internal Medicine residency. I was now 30, just starting my first job, and already being encouraged to think about retirement.

As I matured in my practice and got to know my patients, the subject of their retirement would come up. I was quick to offer my advice: save money and have a plan. A hobby would be essential. I would often recount the story from the previous chapter about Robert's retirement from Alice's perspective. When he came home from work she always had dinner ready for him. Now retired, with no hobby, "He became my 'Boss'," Alice cried to me one day.

His favorite meal was spaghetti. One day, while Alice was preparing dinner he came into the kitchen and gave her detailed instructions on how to cook the sauce and how long to cook the spaghetti. She told me, "I threw him out of the kitchen and told him it was my domain and he had to find something else to do." She went on to tell me, "I gave him a choice, 'Get a job or get a divorce'".

Over the years I've observed many of my patients retire successfully and live happy, content, full lives after a life of "working." But I also learned that retirement is not for everyone; it is perfectly alright to work until you die, *if that is what turns you on*.

Sam became a patient of mine when he was 70. I was on call taking unassigned patients who needed admission through the hospital ER. I thought it odd that Sam, a Benefactor to the hospital, did not have a physician. As far as he was concerned, he just suffered with back pain and "there was nothing anyone could do about it anyway." He was in the ER because he was short of breath and did not know why. Turned out he had untreated hypertension and, as a result, was suffering congestive heart failure. In addition he had been a cigarette smoker for many years; I discovered he had emphysema, too. After a brief admission to the hospital, I treated him (mainly for these three conditions) for the next 20 years, working the magic of modern medicine to control his pain and keep him out of the hospital. Sam was polite but never easy. He had a mind of his own. He was a successful businessman and had been buying up real estate in the Clearwater area for many years, amassing a substantial portfolio. He was working when we met and continued to work until his last week of life, when he was 92. As he explained to me many times, "This is what I love and is all I want to do."

I teased him one day, saying, "All you really want to do is go to the office, open the curtains and look out over your properties." His office was on the top floor of a tall building. He was not ashamed to admit it was true.

"I am turned on by what I have accumulated over the years, but I prefer to have my driver take me right up to the properties so I can look at them up close." Sam was an example to me of someone who believed "If you do something you love, you'll never work a day in your life."

Sam was a man who wanted to maintain control of his life. He was a bit of a handful, a little child stuck in an old man's body. Although his family did everything imaginable to reduce his burdens, he frequently refused. He did develop a great relationship with his massage therapist. He *would* listen to her advice from time to time; she was studying to become a psychologist so she might have had an edge. Getting him to accept help in his home was impossible. He would say, "They just sit around and don't do anything anyway, so why bother."

Getting him to relinquish his driving privileges was another story altogether. He tried to work his charm on me one day by saying, "Doctor, what's the problem with me driving 5 miles to my office?" I responded by exclaiming, "Sam, what is the cop going to see when he pulls you over for speeding: a skinny old man attached to an oxygen tank who needs a walker to walk 5 feet. Besides, how will you ever change your flat tire if you get one?" He thought it over; that conversation led to the end of his driving. Fortunately for Sam, he could afford a driver.

Sam was a puzzle. He worked up until I hospitalized him for the last time. While trying to figure out what might have precipitated his decline, I asked him several questions. His answers were most telling about his life. He was a man of routine. He would wake up and eat the "usual" breakfast, which he prepared himself. At 9:00 a.m., his driver would pick him up and they would start with a brief argument surrounding his refusal to take his portable oxygen with him. The driver would always prevail on this one. He would get to his desk, evaluate his accounts and receipts, pay his bills and be ready to leave. On one of his last trips home, the driver (who was probably paid less than $10 an hour) asked Sam if he was interested in having a burger. Sam loved Wendy's double stacked and agreed. After placing the order, the driver paid for both meals. I asked Sam why, with all his money, he had let the driver pay? He said, "It was his idea to stop." Sam later admitted that when he learned the driver was a Little League coach, he gave him lime to line the base paths with.

Sam's body continued to fail and I was out of miracles. At 92, all Sam's body parts stopped working and he died peacefully, at home. He never retired.

Roy became a patient early in my career. He was the same age as my father, so we had a special bond. It didn't hurt that he grew up in similar circumstances to my father in a section of the lower east side of New York City, the Jewish ghetto of the time. Roy loved sprinkling Yiddish expressions into the conversation during our visits. His favorite was, "Zai Gezuhnt, and all the rest is Bulls**t." He had worked in New York for a number of years, eventually owning and managing slum real estate. He said he enjoyed his tenants and found that they helped him better understand human nature. While Roy had plenty of formal education, he clearly learned a lot about people from his interactions. Our bond intensified when I became his wife's physician. He appreciated the good care I gave her, and they became as grateful as anyone could when I found a small colon cancer on routine cancer screening. She was saved from what would have been a certain and painful death.

Shortly after "retiring" and moving to Florida, Roy realized that there would be bloodshed if he hung around the house with his wife all day. He was lucky: he found part time work, a 20-minute drive from his home.

The Bellevue Biltmore Hotel was a decaying national landmark and hired him as a security guard. "They got a bargain; I am smart. I understand people, and I am loyal." The hotel changed owners several times over the years, but they kept Roy. "I was the only one who really knew what was going on there." Even though he was aging, he was still able to do his job well, and year after year he'd get a raise in his salary. "They know a good thing when they see it," he would say, referring to the management's satisfaction with him and the work he did. I would ask, "Roy, why not retire?" He would give the same answer every time. "Work keeps me alive." And so it has. Four days a week he drives 20 minutes down Alternate US 19, a beautiful costal road with a splendid view of the Gulf and amazing sunsets at night. He gets treated with respect and admiration, and has an opportunity to kibitz with the hotel guests and staff. The job pumps energy and life into his otherwise aged body.

Last week when I was rounding in the hospital I ran into my patient Beverly Davenport. She greeted me with a warm friendly smile as I acknowledged her new bright blue shirt that all the hospital volunteers had recently switched to. Beverly was proud of the multiple jobs she performed as a hospital volunteer. She was carrying a small scrapbook that her fellow volunteers made for her and she allowed me to peruse it. It was an eye-opening experience. As I do with all patients in my practice, I take a social history, that includes work experience but apparently I had forgotten what she had done earlier in her life. Her scrapbook told it all. She had been a second grade teacher for 35 years before retiring and also taught piano "on the side" for a number of years—all while raising her family.

When she and her husband retired to Florida, they both became community volunteers. Not only does she volunteer in the hospital three mornings a week, she also reads to children at a local elementary school and plays golf two days a week. "I love all my volunteer work. I have never been happier," she told me. "Don't get me wrong, I loved teaching too," she added.

The parallel stories of these four individuals reveal that there are multiple ways to enjoy the "golden years." As people are living longer lives, the traditional concept of retirement, which implied the complete abandonment of work, no longer applies. We must now look at retirement as a shift in our life/work balance; moving from a career and raising a family toward enjoying personal leisure and interests while maintaining financial security.

What I have observed (and what these stories illustrate) is that work plays more than just a monetary role in our lives. It helps us feel connected within society. It gives us a focus for some of our energy. It helps us feel a sense of worth and value, and sometimes it is our identity. What people come to realize is that the ideal situation is a balance of work and leisure with the shift moving heavily into leisure (if we can afford it). If we have our health and if we have developed leisure activities, we can greatly enjoy old age.

Money clearly plays a role. For some people, working a shorter work week or having a flexible schedule is conducive to an ideal balance. The uncertainties in the world economy, social security, and the cost of living all make it difficult to anticipate one's future economic needs. With increasing life expectancies, saving enough money to be able to live 20, 30 or 40 years after retirement is daunting. Supplementing retirement income from other sources, perhaps by working part time, can help make "retirement" more comfortable for some.

Today's business environment has begun to appreciate the knowledge and contribution that older workers bring to the workforce. Jobs that require physical strength or dexterity will be staffed by healthier more vibrant individuals, but there is no reason that an older individual cannot make substantial contributions in less strenuous positions to almost any business well into their 70s and, for some individuals, even longer.

Notes on Living Longer

- Retirement is not for everyone. Ask yourself what brings you joy in life.

- Working into old age can provide a purpose and even set positive examples for others.

- Being able to interact with younger people promotes aging with dignity and joy.

- Plan ahead so you can afford retirement.

- Develop hobbies and other interests early in life that you'll be able to continue as you age.

- Find things and people you love and keep them in your day to day plans.
- Maintain strong family bonds that you can enjoy in retirement.
- Develop healthy habits early in life that can be continued into retirement. They will enrich and lengthen your days.
- Improved fitness will result in a longer working career or a longer, healthier retirement.

Resources and Links:

Hansen, Randall S.(2012, April) _Working Beyond Retirement: For Money, Identity, and Purpose._ Retrieved May 2012 from www.quintcareers.com/working_beyond_retirement.html

Joerres, Jeffrey (2009, April) _Aging Your Work Force, Keeping Aging Employees will help Maintain Success._ Retrieved November, 2011 from Todays Wall Street Journal Europe, from http://online.wsj.com/article/SB123923040617102867.html

Maestas, Nicole (2010, July) _Encouraging Work at Older Ages._ A testimony before the Committee on Finance, US Senate. Retrieved January, 2012 from http://rand.org/pubs/testimonies/CT350/

Parker-Pope, Tara (2009, October) _For a Healthy Retirement, Keep Working,_ NYTimes.com. Retrieved November 6, 2011from http://well.blogs.nytimes.com/.../for-a-healthy-retirement-keep-working

The New Definition of Retirement. Retrieved April 22, 2012 from http://Enjoying Retirement.com/HomeRetireDef.asp

Knowledge@Wharton (2010,December) *An End to the 'Golden Years': Increasing Longevity Changes the Work-leisure Equation.* Retrieved April 4, 2011 from http://knowledge.wharton.upenn.edu/article.cfm?articleid=2643

Working to a ripe old age. Retrieved from - National Post www.nationalpost.com/Working+ripe/4377530/story.html - Canada

Chapter 3

100th Birthdays

There is still no cure for the common birthday.
– **John Glenn**

You know you are getting old when the candles cost more than the cake.
– **Bob Hope**

Age is an issue of mind over matter. If you don't mind, it doesn't matter.
– **Mark Twain**

I intend to live forever, or die trying.
– **Groucho Marx**

Throughout the world, longer life expectancy is increasing the number of people in the over-age-65 population. The fastest growing subset of this group that proves the most interesting for researchers are those over age 85, and in particular, the centenarians born in the early 1900s. These individuals lived through the 1918 flu pandemic, saw the birth of the automobile, experienced the Great

Depression and two World Wars, witnessed the assassinations of a President and an American civil rights leader, and watched the first moon landing. They suffered along with all others the fall and devastation of the Twin Towers and attack on the Pentagon—horrific terrorist acts that murdered thousands of innocent civilians on American soil. Throughout their lifetimes, they have seen breakthroughs in the treatment of serious illnesses and watched as AIDS became an epidemic. They have been the first generation to have telephones, movies, radios, televisions, watch the New York Mets win a World Series, experience the development of computers, the Internet and email, and have even survived reality TV. They have followed world events including the election of the nation's first African-American President and Middle East conflicts that appear to have no end in a complex and changing world that each day overwhelms. Throughout these and many other world-shaking events, most have stayed resilient and knowledgeable.

Health officials predict that by 2050, more than 800,000 Americans will be pushing into their second century of life. The patients I describe in my anecdotes and the majority of individuals over the age of 85 *are* mentally alert and relatively free of disabilities. They remain active members of their communities. They represent a new model of aging, one that health experts are hoping more of us can emulate—both to make our lives fuller and to ease the inevitable healthcare burden that our longer-living population will impose in coming decades.

As I reflect on the many significant events in my career, some of my most enlightening memories were made when a patient celebrated a 100th birthday.

Pat, Betsey, and Trudy have been patients of mine for at least a dozen years each. These wonderful ladies present the tremendous contrasts in the human experience that I enjoy each and every day as I set out to work.

Pat is a happy person. She has a large and loving family, grew up in the DC area where her father owned a prominent brewery, allowing her to live a life of luxury. Pat had been married to a General in the army and enjoyed the global travel that came with the position. She thoroughly enjoyed raising her children, was devoted to her grandchildren and great-grandchildren, and was a renowned bridge player. Her earliest visits to me focused on the diagnosis and treatment of her Alzheimer's disease. She was always pleasant, witty, and usually flirtatious. While the disease ravaged her short term memory, it did not put a damper on her zest for life. Regardless of how advanced her Alzheimer's Dementia became, Pat remained a fantastic card player and could beat anyone in bridge who dared to play her. She was surrounded by wonderful aides who provided compassionate care to her throughout the years. This allowed her to stay in her own home located in a very exclusive section of Clearwater. Pat was always impeccably dressed and well groomed when she came in for her appointments. She would regularly greet me as though she had never met me before and would start with, "Where am I and what am I doing here?"

In the weeks leading up to her 100th birthday, she developed an inflammation of her elbow, bursitis. It was a challenge to get it resolved. As a result, I saw her weekly for about six weeks. Pat had great big blue eyes that were constantly trying to flirt with me, and her remarks were punctuated with some type of sarcasm or sexual overtone. On one occasion when I asked her to get on the exam table, Pat replied, "Is that all you want me to do?" When I asked her to remove her shirt, she often asked, "Is that all I need to take off?" She was devilish with those seductive bright blue eyes. Had I been closer to her age, I would have been flattered but with a 50 year gap between us, I just chuckled.

It was an honor for me to receive a formal invitation to Pat's 100th birthday party, which was to be held at a classy yacht club on Clearwater Beach. It was my weekend "on call" for my physicians' call group. I took delight in bragging to all the hospital nurses that I was going to my patient's 100th birthday. I felt such great pride when the nurses asked all about this very special patient, and I raved about how extraordinary she was.

When I arrived at the yacht club there must have been more than 100 guests in attendance, including family from all over the US, friends from her bridge club, and military widows. We all circulated around the room and I introduced myself and connected with members of her family. Her son, daughters and even grandchildren knew me by name based on the reports given to them by Pat's caregivers. Each expressed their appreciation for the many issues I had helped Pat with over the years. When the one hour of cocktails and petit fours ended, Pat was given a great big cake with 100 candles all glowing. Pat was about to blow out the candles on the gigantic cake when her son yelled, "Mom make a wish." Pat took a big exaggerated deep breath and blew out all 100 candles. Pat's granddaughter put her arm around her and asked, "Grandma, tell us what your wish was?" I gasped, fearful of the type of remark could come out of her mouth, thinking how embarrassed her family would be if she uttered some off color sexual remarks. Much to my surprise and delight, she said, "I wish for 100 years more." I was astonished that Pat could be so witty, and as her physician, I was thinking that this would be a tall order for me to fill! Family and friends lined up to wish her well. I spent a few minutes just watching her, soaking up the excitement of the event.

Pat and I chatted for a few moments about the experience and what it meant for her to turn 100 years old. She said, "This is the most excitement I have had in years!" She was totally charming and alive. One week later, at a return visit to my office, I inquired about her birthday party, and sadly she did not recall one minute of it. She didn't even remember that she had turned 100 years old. I showed her the picture I took of her with my cell phone and she exclaimed, "Is that me? My, I look very pretty in that picture." What I can say about Pat is that she has been pleasantly confused, happy and lived a good and full life. When asked about her life, she reflected and said, "I have no regrets about anything."

The next patient of mine to turn 100 was Betsey. She celebrated her 100th birthday at my office with my staff after I had completed examining her on a routine office visit. It was no coincidence that her special day occurred on the day she was to have a scheduled time with me. We had been her support system, and there was no one else for her to celebrate with. The funny thing was that when she arrived, she asked, "Why do I have an appointment today? There is nothing wrong with me today." For the previous 20 visits Betsey had *something* wrong: her neck, her head, her nerves, her heart, or was it her stomach? Today, nothing was wrong so she said, "Why am I here, Doctor?" I simply told her that Medicare was paying for her birthday visit today. (I was just kidding her; Medicare does not pay for birthday visits.) She responded with a bashful grin and told me, "You did not have to do that for me." Little did she know I was doing it for me. Maybe I wanted to attend as many 100th birthday parties as I could and be in the Guinness Book of Records one day.

Betsey was born in Scotland in 1907 and endured WWI as a child and WWII as a young woman. She remembered the bombings from the German Luftwaffe of the port town in which she lived in the 1940s. She recalled many of the details of her life before and after she arrived in the United States. During our lunch together Betsey told me, "My brothers came to the US and worked in a quarry in Ohio, raising enough money to be able to sponsor the rest of her family to make the trip to the States. I married an Englishman but we had no children. I worked as a clerk and got divorced from my husband after about 10 years. He was a nice man but he was an alcoholic, and the marriage was not a good one. When my sister became a widow we moved in together and were nearly inseparable for over 30 years." They lived in a small "villa" in a subsidized retirement community. During one visit she shared something we all take for granted: how she and her sister performed their grocery shopping. Once a week they would compile a short list of items they regularly bought: milk, coffee, and fruit. Promptly at ten o'clock on Tuesdays, Betsey (97 years old at the time) and her older sister, Agnes (98), would wait outside their residence for a "surrey" from their facility to pick them up and drive them two miles to the Publix grocery store. The surrey would depart Publix at precisely eleven o'clock providing them just one hour to accomplish their shopping. The surrey driver would help them load the one or two bags of groceries and return the women to their villa. Betsey and Agnes would work together placing the items in the cupboard or refrigerator. Imagine, two women in their late 90's taking a bus to the local grocery store to shop. What an unbelievable feat, but as Betsey explained to me, "It was just another of the daily chores we had been doing all our lives, so why stop now?"

At age 98, Agnes died after an episode of diverticulitis. Betsey was devastated, as Agnes was all she had. For the next three years when Betsey was lonely, one of her many symptoms would crop up precipitating an office visit. I rarely found anything I could fix. I would offer her a pain pill, an antidepressant, physical therapy, but I found she mostly just wanted to talk or get something off her chest.

For Betsey, living to be 100 was not the blessing that it has been for Pat. She had no surviving family, and as a result my office staff and I were her family. While Pat viewed her glass as half full, Betsey saw hers as half empty. Even as she approached the century mark she was bothered by the little things. For example, one day she was beside herself when she observed that the staff at her facility had a small party and despite cleaning up their mess, they had left a few glasses on a table. "This is my home, Doctor, and they have no business leaving a mess like that!"

The year after Betsey turned 100, two more patients celebrated their centennials and again I had the good fortune to share time with them. One of these patients was Trudy, who celebrated her 100th birthday with my staff and me much like Betsey had. She had outlived most of her family and friends, so she would spend this special day with us. While Trudy had lived in the same retirement community for the past 18 years, she would have to wait three days to celebrate the event in group fashion with others in her community. I am certain she was the only one that year to celebrate the number 100.

My office staff and I look forward to these celebrations of 100 years of life. Our planning starts about one year ahead when we try to jog office visits in such a way that the birthdays fall on the exact day of an appointment. My staff practice scrapbooking as a hobby and their role is taking pictures of the event and using them to create a personalized scrapbook to commemorate it. When we schedule the party, we ask our special guest to order a favorite lunch. We can have it on hand as part of the celebration. As our staff gathered around, Trudy was served the roast beef sandwich she had requested. Ever the independent one, Trudy carefully prepared to eat her sandwich by opening and spreading mayonnaise from an aluminum packet. As she performed this task, I realized that the condiment packet was an invention, like many others, that had come along late in her lifetime, one that we take for granted as an ordinary convenience of life. As she took her first bite of the roast beef sandwich, I began asking her questions. In retrospect it might have been somewhat impolite to hit her with a barrage of questions before she even finished her first bite of that delicious roast beef sandwich. Although I had known her for 18 years and knew a lot about her, it was meaningful to me for my staff to get to know and experience this remarkable woman as she celebrated the centennial year of her life. She was a great example for my staff and had lessons to share with all of us. I started out with, "Trudy, when and where were your born?" I corrected myself, realizing she was 100 years old and added, "I know you were born in 1909." Trudy answered with a distinct and thick New York accent, "I was born in Brooklyn, New York, and grew up in the Prospect Park section," she answered. We talked for a bit about what Brooklyn was like so long ago. "Nothing like it is now," she added, "it was beautiful, with open fields, not the concrete jungle and crime-filled area it is today." She grew up before Coney Island and the famous roller coaster, "The Cyclone," had been built. She recalled that this landmark attraction had opened in 1927. As I tried to get her to recollect memories from the past, I casually asked her who the President was at the time. I was taken aback by her response as jokingly she replied, "What is this, a quiz or something?" I got the hint and backed off before guessing, "Warren G. Harding?" No one bothered to correct the boss, but the correct answer was William Howard Taft.

We did not talk much about her family, but I can assume that they suffered through the Great Depression much like everyone else in that generation. I inquired about her education and she told me, "I graduated from public high school and went on to Business College." It was there that she learned a trade, which allowed her to work in an office, typing and taking shorthand. She told me that her boss was out of the office much of the time so she had many different responsibilities. She had really enjoyed her job and prospered. She never married.

I asked her to tell me about the most adventurous event she could remember in her life. Without much hesitation she said, "Ice skating on a lake in Prospect Park." I asked if it had anything to do with social interaction and meeting boys. She laughed. "No. We were always afraid that the ice had not completely frozen and we were afraid that we would fall in."

"Trudy," I asked, "what about that story you told me about your trip to Cuba in the mid-50s?" A few years earlier, I had begun asking my patients unscripted questions to gain insight to understand their lives. Trudy was my very first victim. I had asked her what the most exciting event of her life was. She gazed up at me with her adoring blue eyes and said, "I don't know." I pressed her again for an answer and before she could give me the same reply, I took a wild guess and said, "You went skinny dipping." Much to my surprise she replied, "How did you guess?" That was a moment that neither of us would ever forget. She recalled, "My friends and I had been on vacation at the National Hotel in Cuba before the revolution. We snuck into the pool late at night and frolicked for about two hours." When I asked what made them stop, she said, "The hotel security chased us out, but what a great time we all had!" I was thrilled when she retold the entire story of her trip to Cuba to our staff, as I thought it was one of the better stories I have heard in my career as a physician.

My partner in my medical practice, Ben, always one to stir up controversy, asked the next question, "Trudy, what has been the secret to your long life?" Her answer was short and simple, "I like to eat liver and onions." We all had a chuckle. I teased her about the secret to her long life by reminding her and my staff that she had never been married, and she agreed *that* might have been another reason for her longevity.

Our lunchtime party concluded with a chorus of "Happy Birthday" for the 100ᵗʰ time in her life. She blew out the one candle on her cake, cut the cake and ate her piece like a teenager. Our party ended when her ride arrived to take her back to her retirement community. We all felt so fortunate to have shared these rare but valuable moments with this centenarian.

What have I learned from celebrating birthdays with 100 year olds? First, it seems like there are more 100 year old women than men. Second, when you live to be 100, you are likely to outlive your spouse and siblings, and endure events that often lead to sadness, loss and grief.

Most people today fall prey to chronic diseases that strike in mid to late life—conditions such as cancer, heart disease, stroke and dementia—and end up nursing disabilities stemming from these illnesses for the remainder of their lives. Centenarians, on the other hand, appear to be remarkably resilient when it comes to shrugging off such ailments; they seem to draw on some reserve that allows them to bounce back from health problems and remain relatively hearty until their final days. Dozens of studies have investigated such individuals, with the goal of discovering the secrets to their salubrious seniority. Those analyses, however, have generally followed two separate if parallel tracks. The traditional approach has been to study the lifestyle and behavioral components of vigorous aging—the good habits, such as a healthy diet, regular physical activity and mental exercises that might keep the elderly vibrant through their golden years. The New England Centenarian Study, which includes 850 people entering their 100s, for example, has identified several behavioral and personality traits that seem to be critical to longevity, including: not smoking, being extroverted and easygoing, and staying lean.

Japanese studies have shown five factors that have contributed to the large number of centenarians in a coastal region:

1. A diet that is heavy on grains, fish, and vegetables and light on meat, eggs, and dairy products.
2. Low-stress lifestyles, which are proven significantly less stressful than that of the mainland inhabitants of Japan, for example.
3. A caring community, where older adults are not isolated and are taken better care of.
4. High levels of activity, where locals work until an older age than the average age in other countries, and where there is more emphasis on activities like walking and gardening to keep active.
5. Spirituality, where a sense of purpose comes from involvement in spiritual matters and prayer eases the mind of stress and problems.

Although these factors vary from those mentioned in the previous study, the culture of Okinawa has proven these aspects to be important in its large population of centenarians.

Even if you associate with younger people throughout your life, if you live to be 100 you are still likely to outlive most of your friends and companions. In addition, if your friends have family in another geographic area, their family is likely to insist on relocating them or will place them in a different long-term care setting, thus adding to the many possibilities that would result in loss of a relationship.

While I have a firm belief that genetics plays a crucial role in how we age, good habits and good luck must also play a role. Eating right, remaining active mentally and physically were clearly present in the lives of the three patients I have described here. Being in the right place at the right time is also important. These women did not participate in risky behavior (unless you consider skinny dipping in pre-revolution Cuba as risky). Each one of them or their families saw to it that as they aged they remained in safe, structured environments that provided them just the right amount of services they needed and allowed as much independence as possible. It seems that their ability to remain independent might have played a major role in their will to survive, for if it was absent they might have lost the will to live.

Notes for living longer

- Living to be 100 years of age is a confluence of genes, luck, and attitude.
- With scientific discoveries and progress in health care more and more adults will live to be 100 years old.
- Maintain a positive attitude about life; if you have a bad attitude, living a long life can be miserable.
- If you wish to live to be 100, live a sensible life: reduce your risks, lower your stress level, and follow healthy habits.
- Maintain connections to family and friends especially those younger than you. They will keep you active, vibrant and will be your support later in life.
- Ask your doctor to help you work toward *quality* of life and not just longevity.

Resources and Links:

K8 N (2009, October) *Centenarian-Secrets.* Retrieved October 3, 2011from http://k8n.hubpages.com/hub/Centenarian-Secrets

NY Times (2010, October) *Secrets of the Centenarians, Life Before, During and After 100.* Retrieved August 27, 2012 from http://www.nytimes.com/interactive/2010/10/19/health/20101018-centenarians-voices-photos.html

Health Checkup: How to Live 100 Years

A century of life was once a rare thing, but that is changing. Science is slowly unraveling the secrets of the centenarians

Oz, Mehmet (2010, Feb) *Living Long and Living Well.* Retrieved August 8, 2011 from http://www.time.com/time/special/packages/article/,28804,1963392_1963369_1963380,00.html

Chapter 4

Birth Certificates Don't Matter
Goals, adventure, and attitudes

You don't stop laughing because you grow old.
You grow old because you stop laughing.
– **Michael Pritchard**

The longer I live the more beautiful life becomes.
– **Frank Lloyd Wright**

We do not stop playing because we grow old;
we grow old because we stop playing.
– **Benjamin Franklin**

One of the expected benefits I have derived from the practice of medicine is that it often places me at the intersection of my personal life and my patients' experiences. I have been allowed to view my experiences in life through the lives of my patients, using each one to deepen the meaning of my life. Similarly, I have shared my life's encounters with my patients to assist them on their life journey.

Many situations with my own family are included in this book as they have served as an important backdrop to perspectives I share with my patients. One such example involves my two sons.

I'm very proud of my boys and have always had pictures of them displayed prominently throughout my medical office. I've found that patients want to relate to their physicians as people. These photographs show that I am more than a doctor—I have a family. (I believe the pictures also help when I am just not available to patients because I am spending time with my family.) There are two particular pictures of my sons that I keep in my office that serve as examples of some of the traits I see in some very special patients.

One is a picture of my younger son, Jake, from his Little League days; he was about 9 years old at the time and he was set to field a ball while playing 3rd base. While he had always been an outgoing child with lots of friends, he did not let their fears or concerns have a negative influence him. One example of his concentration was that as he fielded balls hit to him at 3rd base he would think only about what he saw when he watched major leaguers on TV. What he observed from these games was this: when the ball was hit to the fielder he would pick it up and throw it to first base. Jake never considered the potential to make an error and with this attitude he became proficient as a fielder. On the other hand, the other boys who had negative thoughts about making errors would commit errors, a thought that never crossed Jake's mind.

My older son, Chad, has a different personality and the picture of him hanging in my office is also very symbolic. I took it in his senior year of high school at his last "at bat" of the season and I will always remember the moment. It had been a difficult season for him; he was unhappy with the amount of playing time he was getting and he had contemplated quitting the team. There were at least two reasons though that he remained. His close friends from school were on the team and he really enjoyed being with them. The second reason was that he never quit anything. Had he quit, I would never have gotten this very meaningful picture and he might not have seen the clear message that one doesn't quit or stop doing what they have always done when faced with adversity.

Susan is a patient of mine who demonstrates an attitude that there are no obstacles in life. Since her husband passed away two years prior, she became a volunteer clown at the hospital and was an active member of the Red Hats. Once a month she sings with a group of women called "Sweet Adelines" and has returned to playing golf a few times a week—when she can fit it into her busy schedule.

She was 86 years old when she was in my office recently telling me she just spent 11 days out of town and did not make one single "mistake." When I inquired what she was talking about, she elaborated.

"I flew from Clearwater to St. Louis, rented a car with GPS and drove to the middle of Missouri to attend my deceased husband's class reunion. I spent 9 additional days following a plan, visiting various family member and old friends, along with visits to several museums before returning home." She was so proud that she had accomplished this without making a mistake, she was exuberant. Then she said, "It was no big deal, Doc, it was just like so many trips Ed and I had always taken."

Well, I considered it an amazing accomplishment. Imagine what this 86 year old woman had to do. She had to read her mail, commit ahead of time to attend the reunion and then map out her trip including plans to visit others along the way. She had to book airline tickets and reserve a rental car. She had to arrange her medications for the trip, pack for all 11 days, and plan for many changes of clothes. She needed to arrange to get to the airport with enough time to get through security not to mention traverse her way to the gate when she would board the plane. After a two-hour flight, this 86-year-old woman—with arthritis in all her joints—would get off the plane all by herself and make her way to the rental car agency with all her luggage and then drive two hours to the middle of Missouri! That trip would exhaust any 50 year old! I could not imagine the effects a trip like that would have on a woman of her age. After 11 days, she had returned home, "with a sense of accomplishment and pride." Her resilience, focus, and her "no big deal" attitude speaks volumes about her adventurous attitude. I envy her attitude and hope to follow her example as I age.

I had a similar experience recently with a new patient named Millie. Millie became one of my favorite patients in a short period of time. She was a snowbird from the suburbs outside Detroit, Michigan. I am not certain how she got my name to become my patient, but her daughter is a physician in Michigan and she may have researched my credentials beforehand. The first time Millie visited me at my office, she was 87 and experiencing extremely high blood pressure. She brought her husband with her. She had been to the ER the prior evening and had been given an additional medication in an attempt to get her blood pressure down. Millie could not understand what was causing this, and inquired, "Why the heck is my blood pressure so high, Doctor?"

I must have asked her 100 questions, grilling her like she was under the lights at a police station in a 1950s detective movie. "What was your pressure last week and last month? What did you eat the day before your pressure went up? Did you recently switch to a generic brand of medication or perhaps miss one dose?"

Her answers did not help me understand her situation any better. Then her husband said, "Millie, tell him about your back pain. Maybe that has something to do with it?" She looked at him like he was crazy and then said," I have been having a severe pain in my back. Is there any relationship between that and my blood pressure?" "Not as far as I can tell," I replied, "but are you taking any medication for your back pain?"

"No doctor, but I have been applying a cream my physician up North gave me."

I had been about to start a new line of questioning. "What type of cream are you applying?"

"Voltaren gel," she replied.

I was taken by surprise as this is a gel to be applied only to joints and she was applying it to a muscle sprain. I looked at her with a quizzical glance and asked her, "What joint had it been prescribed for?"

"My doctor told me to apply it to a small area on my back where I have a small cyst and it pushes on my sciatic nerve." Now my expression changed to one of disbelief; she and her husband noticed and become concerned. I try to keep my poker face on during situations like this but I had difficulty controlling myself. Voltaren has been available in tablet form for many years and I am well aware that it can elevate a person's blood pressure but I have never seen this with any of my patients. My best judgment at the time was that the Voltaren gel was the culprit and so (figuring that is what I get paid the big bucks for), I told her that's what I thought. I gave her some reassurance, and sent her home. I instructed her to check her blood pressure daily for the next few days and report back to me early the following week. She and her husband walked slowly out of my office in a mild state of disbelief. Millie called the very next day to report the miracle: her blood pressure had returned to normal and that she just could not believe that the Voltaren gel could have had that effect!   Two days later she was back in my office praising me for recognizing the cause of her blood pressure elevation and then pleading, "Please, fix my aching back!"

I had just accomplished a major feat by getting her blood pressure down and now she wanted me to eliminate the pain in her 87-year-old back. Since she was a new patient I was at a disadvantage and had no idea what caused her back pain. I started my detective work all over again. I could tell just by looking at her that she was in severe pain, and 87 year old women don't exaggerate their pain. First I thought she might have a compression fracture from a fall but she denied any such event. Next I thought it could be her mattress, and on and on I went without success. Her husband politely interrupted, "Millie, what about the dancing we did the other night at the Italian club?"

Millie sharply replied, "Don't be ridiculous, we have been dancing every Friday night for the past 25 years, how could that be the cause?" My jaw dropped when I discovered that this couple danced every week. Millie added, "Yes, dance is what has kept us fit and is a way we connect with each other at least once a week, and it *is* great fun. I could never hurt myself dancing."

I was just about to agree with her about the health benefits of dancing when her husband interjected, "Millie, what about the dance you did with Phillip?"

"What are you implying? We just had one dance, and it was perfectly innocent" she retorted.

"I was referring to the type of dance you did, the Meringue," he responded.

"Oh, how could that ever hurt my back?" she said. Just then she stood up and demonstrated the Meringue. She began to swivel her hips as if she was dancing with her friend Phillip and suddenly she grabbed her back, looked at me, and immediately all three of us knew why her back hurt! We had figured it out. My course of treatment was physical therapy. Three weeks later she was back dancing again, but understood the Meringue put too much strain on the hips and it was banned from her dance card.

During a quiet time in my office surrounded by pictures of my family and travels, I had time to reflect about the patients in the previous stories and the significance they have to aging and longevity.

What Susan accomplished was remarkable and courageous; I was very proud of her. How did she accomplish this? She did what my son Jake did, she gave herself positive messages: that traveling to Missouri was something she had done in the past and there were no obstacles in the present. Although she did not admit it to me, she must have tired at some point, but then she did what my son Chad demonstrated to me: she stayed in the game, she did not quit. Chad, Jake and Susan got their rewards when they achieved their goals. Susan shows no signs of giving up or giving in to the date on her birth certificate.

Millie is an example of how older people can dance their way to improved health and happiness as documented in many studies done all over the world. In 2009, The Journal of Aging and Physical Activity reported a study that demonstrated the potential for dancing to improve physical functioning in older adults. The study revealed improved aerobic conditioning, lower body muscle endurance, strength and flexibility, static and dynamic balance/agility and gait speed in older, especially female, adults.

Another conclusion in the study was that dancing provides older adults another physical activity option that might improve their all-around physical capability. A well-documented benefit of dancing is the continued engagement in life, which aids in successful aging. It contributes to longevity by giving adults something to enjoy and focus on and look forward to. It alleviates social isolation and can take away aches and pains (unless you are doing the Meringue with Phil!) of aging. Dancing can be attributed to the enhanced connection between aging adults and enhancing relationships. In addition it can be viewed as a social event that enhances connections with others in one's community.

Like my son Jake, Millie did not have a preconceived notion of what she could not do or when she had to stop dancing. There was no sign outside the dance hall restricting people by their age. In addition, like my son Chad, who participated in sports to be with his friends, Millie danced because she shared this activity with her husband, Phil, and their other friends, seeking to maintain connections.

Susan and Millie are just two of my patients with remarkable stories that I have had the privilege to treat over my 30 years in practice of medicine. They show no regard for the date printed on their birth certificates, going about life without the limitations others set on age. It is a beautiful and inspiring thing to observe.

Notes on living longer

- Age has no bearing on what you can accomplish if you have the desire.
- A positive attitude will help overcome physical limitations.

- Know your personal limitations but do not let them be dictated by your age.
- If you can dream it, you can do it.
- It is appropriate to ask for help when necessary.

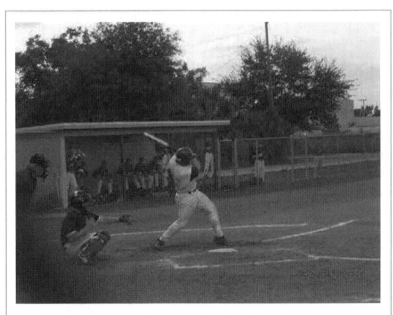

MY SON CHAD GETTING A HIT IN HIS LAST
HIGH SCHOOL AT BAT

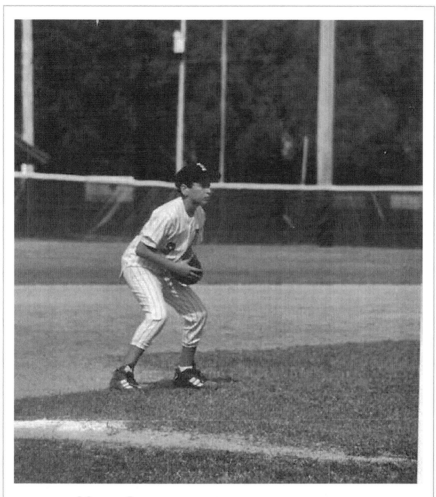

MY SON JACOB CONCENTRATING WHILE WAITING
TO FIELD A GROUND BALL

Chapter 5

Gratitude
Hitting Singles and Home Runs

*Kind words can be short and easy to speak, but
their echoes are truly endless*

– Mother Teresa

Susan and Millie demonstrate what we would all consider a positive, go-getter attitude, but there are other attitudes that have favorable effects as well. Having a sense of gratitude as a state of mind can lead to greater fulfillment and a more satisfying life. We can interpret one of the Ten Commandments, "Thou shall not covet thy neighbor or thy neighbor's wife," as an instruction to be grateful for what we have. In her song "Soak up the Sun", Sheryl Crow sings, "It's not having what you want; it's wanting what you've got."

Practicing Internal Medicine and Geriatrics is rarely glamorous or sexy, and there is little immediate gratification. For the most part I spend my day treating chronic medical problems such as diabetes, high blood pressure, and high cholesterol. Most of my patients have multiple medical problems, so you can add to this list: arthritis, heart failure, depression, insomnia, and Alzheimer's disease. I also manage the care of patients at the end of their lives, providing them an opportunity to make heroic and difficult decisions as they face death. I find these encounters both challenging and rewarding. This work is emotional and stressful, and it is not like hitting a home run. There is no immediate reward for reducing someone's blood pressure from 180 to 120, however, I have had the opportunity of hitting a home run every now and again, and in those cases I am as grateful and appreciative as my patients.

One such patient was Millicent, 62 at the time when she came to my office alarmed after she noted blood in her toilet bowl after she had a bowel movement. After I took a detailed history about her condition, I examined her and scheduled her to have an in office sigmoidoscopy for the following day. This is a procedure I learned long ago, in my medical training, and it allows the doctor to view inside the lower portion of a patient's colon. It's an excellent way to look for causes of bleeding, including colon cancers. The scope typically used in a primary care office is 60cm (over 2 feet) long, much shorter than the scope used for a colonoscopy. The sigmoidoscopy does not require that the patient be put to sleep. I had performed this procedure in my office until the United States Public Health Task Force on screening tests along with the American College of Gastroenterology and the National Cancer Institute, reported that a colonoscopy performed every 10 years had a greater success for detecting colon cancer.

During Millicent's sigmoidoscopy exam, I found a mass in her lower colon. This was my first encounter with this type of finding. I was fairly new at the procedure and was startled when I saw the mass. It appeared to be large, and looked like a walnut shell spray-painted fire engine red. It was clearly abnormal and probably cancerous. I performed a biopsy and expected the pathology report to confirm my suspicion of colon cancer. A week later I called Millicent into my office to discuss the findings and make recommendations.

Millicent arrived for her appointment with her husband, Roy. They were seated in my office when I sat down behind my desk and opened her chart. Roy was a bit nervous but was calm in comparison to his wife. Millicent was well-dressed but reeked of tobacco and coffee. She thought that, at age 62, she was too old to have an operation and her body language matched her demeanor.

"Good morning, Millicent," I started as I looked up from her chart, "and good morning to you, Roy. I appreciate you both coming in today. I would like to discuss the report of your biopsy, Millicent." I noted their anxiety so my intention was to get right to the point.

"Good morning, Dr. Bernstein," Roy chimed in. "Please forgive Millicent as she is a very nervous person and is quite tense about this biopsy report."

"Roy, I will do the talking for myself. I am a grown up," Millicent interrupted. "Besides, it doesn't matter because I am not doing anything about it. I am done with testing and there will be no surgery. I am too old. Let me enjoy the time I have left."

"Millicent, just listen to the man," Roy asserted.

"Millicent," I interjected, "with all due respect, allow me to just tell you the result first and then I will add my interpretation of what it means before you jump to any conclusions."

"OK," she replied. "I will behave myself—for a little while." She sat up in her chair as if she were a school girl who had just been scolded by her teacher.

I started, "The lesion I biopsied was cancerous, and based on its size it needs to be surgically removed."

"Doctor," Millicent interrupted. "Don't forget, I am 62 years old and I'm a smoker. Doesn't that exclude me as a surgical candidate?"

"Millicent," I responded. "I am well aware of your age and the fact that you have been smoking cigarettes for nearly 50 years will present some obstacles, but I feel you are fit enough for surgery. I actually believe that if the cancer is confined to a small segment of your colon, you will be cured when it is removed."

"But, Doctor," Millicent replied. "I haven't been a patient in a hospital since I gave birth to my second daughter 45 years ago."

I started to think, *Here I am with a chance to make a huge difference in this patient's life —hit a home run—and she is resisting me! I cannot let her get away.* I needed to come up with something profound that would persuade her. "Millicent," I sighed, "this is the kind of cancer that will grow slowly, be very painful and, eventually, kill you. It will leave your husband a widower. Look at him; he will never be able to survive without you."

"I will need a few days to consider my options," Millicent added.

"Don't worry, Doc," Roy interrupted with a wink, "when our daughters and I get through with her, she will be back here ready for surgery."

The next day my office manager, Vicki, tapped me on the shoulder and said, "What did you say to Millicent the other day? She just called and wants to know which surgeon you want her to see to for the mass in her colon?"

After my remarks and with a little persuasion from her husband and daughters, Millicent had the lower part of her colon removed. That was more than 20 years ago and she has not had a recurrence of cancer since.

Each time she comes for an office visit, which is about every 3 months, she reminds me how grateful she is that I performed the sigmoidoscopy. She understands that she would have eventually died an early and painful death if she had declined my recommendation at the time. Her melodrama in thanking me makes me feel good. It reminds me of the two home runs I hit: one while performing her sigmoidoscopy, and the second when I convinced her to have the operation. Perhaps for the rest of my days treating patients, I will just be hitting singles.

Another patient who is comfortable expressing gratitude was Bob. He was 60 years old, retired from the Merchant Marines, when he came to see me for the first time. He had spent much of his career in the Panama Canal region before settling in Dunedin, Florida. As he established himself in my office for his medical care, I prepared to initiate a program of preventive screening tests for him. The testing would include a complete blood count work-up, a blood chemistry profile, a cholesterol level, a thyroid blood test, a PSA (prostate cancer screening test) and a sigmoidoscopy. Bob did not resist any of these recommendations and, unlike the struggles I had with Millicent, he was always very cooperative. "You're the Doctor," Bob would always say with a warm and grateful smile.

Since Bob had been a cigarette smoker for many years, he was at risk for the development of coronary artery disease. When his cholesterol level was moderately elevated, it added an additional risk for a heart attack and I placed him on Mevacor® as it was the only statin-cholesterol medication available at the time. On the day he came in to have a sigmoidoscopy, I still had limited experience with this test. During my medical school training, I had studied what colon pathology looked like and could identify it when something looked abnormal, as I had with Millicent. As I inserted the scope, I saw a 2-cm red mushroom shaped polyp. I knew right then and there that it was a colon cancer and had to be removed. Bob was a quiet man and not one for histrionics (unlike Millicent). I sat with him, giving him what amounted to the same news I had given Millicent.

"Doc," Bob responded, "I want to get started right away. Who do you recommend as a surgeon?"

I arranged for Bob to see a colon surgeon for a removal of a portion of the colon. The final pathology report was a Duke B colon cancer (this is *a stage 2* colon cancer—out of a maximum of 4). By undergoing the surgery, he was cured of his colon cancer, and I can tell you he has never forgotten the home run I hit the day I performed his sigmoidoscopy.

Bob had a unique history as far as cancer goes. During the 20 years I cared for him, I had diagnosed skin cancers, a throat cancer, a prostate cancer and, lastly, a non-operable lung cancer. He dealt with each new diagnosis bravely and never forgot to thank me.

The last challenge with Bob was our discussion about his lung cancer. When given the various options for treatments he told me, "Doc, I have lived a good life and I know that there is no treatment that would allow me to live longer." At age 84, Bob explained, "I would prefer not to suffer from the effects of treatments that would not do anything to maintain or improve the quality of my life." As grateful as he has always been for what I had done with my sigmoidoscope, he was equally grateful for the time and emotion I put forth in counseling him about choices for his future.

There can be unexpected expressions of gratitude in my practice as well. At age 85, Pete had been a patient of mine for more than 20 years. When we first met I treated him for severe high blood pressure. It required a lot of savvy on my part to adjust his five medications while attempting to minimize any side effects. When I discovered his high cholesterol, I prescribed medication for management and reductions of dangerous levels. Later, Pete developed diabetes and prostate cancer. I continued to help him manage all the disease processes as well as the embarrassing side effects (urinary incontinence) of his radiation therapy for his prostate cancer. Each visit generally started like this: "Hey, Doc, how is your family?" After I told him what my children were up to, he would say, "Have you been away recently? I just came back from skiing and I know this great place in Utah." (I don't ski, but it made for an interesting conversation.)

I guess we bonded over the years, and I took for granted how much he appreciated what I had done to manage his very complicated regimen of medications and keep his lab work in line. At one point he developed a severe case of shingles (a painful inflammation of the nerves—the visible symptom is a rash—that can occur in those who have had chicken pox earlier in life). Months later, after the rash had cleared up, he still continued to have severe pain in the location where the rash first appeared. This condition is called post herpetic neuralgia. He did not want to take too many narcotics; he had found the side effects unpleasant. While I was telling him about an alternative narcotic to reduce his pain, he turned to me and said, "You know, Doctor, if it weren't for you I wouldn't be around. You have kept me alive much longer than I or anyone in my family would have expected."

In the midst of a very busy day, I was touched by his expression of genuine gratitude. It was heartfelt and spontaneous. He went on to tell me how all the things I had done for him had kept him alive, so that it extended his retirement, allowing him more time to enjoy his family and his life on the beach. His comments lifted my spirits on an otherwise stressful and challenging day. Until then, I had been unaware of how grateful he was for what I considered *"just doing my job!"*

Notes for living longer:

- Gratitude is a state of mind, an emotion or attitude that is distinctly human.
- Within the 10 commandments, "Thou shall not covet thy neighbor or thy neighbor's wife," commands that we be grateful for what we have.
- Sheryl Crow sings, *"It's not having what you want. It's wanting what you've got."*
- Be grateful for every day you have.
- The person to whom you are grateful might not even be aware of it. Share your gratitude; in doing so you will be giving a deeply satisfying gift.
- Show gratitude to those members of your family and friends you care about.
- Express your gratitude to those who help you as they might not be aware of how much you value what they have done.

Resources and Links:

Successful Aging
http://cas.umkc.edu/casww/SA/ResourceRefLinks.htm

Chapter 6

Sex, Denial, and Home Health Aides

The heart that loves is always young
– **Greek Proverb**

As people get older they become more of what they were
– **Rita Bernstein, my mother**

I had just driven across the state of Florida on my way to spend a special weekend with my aging parents. Mom was turning 81 and Dad was 89. Dad had become frail and with each passing day more stubborn and ornery. We had about an hour before we were to leave for dinner with a few close family members. Mom, Dad and I began a familiar refrain about getting assistance for them in their home. Dad needed someone to help him get out of bed and dressed in the morning, and empty his urinal. Mom could no longer get him up and refuses to do the urinal routine. My brother, sister and I have broached the subject many times in the past three years and there is always a reason the aides were not satisfactory.

"She smells, another one doesn't wash her hands," Mom says. "This one is too tall, that one has an annoying laugh," Dad adds. Mom doesn't care for one, Dad doesn't like another.

"Why pay someone to sit around? We don't have that much stuff that needs to be done", they both agree on that one.

In the meantime, Dad is at high risk for a fall, which could eventually lead to a total loss of independence. Mom is so fed up with the man, she sleeps in the other bedroom. They can't agree on who snores louder. She cannot even leave him alone to get some "space." Upon her return she hears a barrage of questions: where had she gone? Why did it take so long and where was his lunch? It has become quite unpleasant for her. "He just doesn't leave me alone," Mom adds with disgust. No one has ever been able to stand up to Dad. As the years have progressed he has gotten more and more difficult. Mom, the great philosopher always says "As people get older they become more of what they truly are." Over the years I have found this kernel of wisdom to be true.

She is talking about her husband; my father. I gave it my best, trying to get some compromise but around and around we went without a commitment to get any home help. The discussion reminded me of one of my favorite lines—about a river in Egypt— De-Nile. After a long discussion, it was time to join the family for dinner.

As I drove to the restaurant, I reflected on another similar family situation, the Horner's. It's best to begin when we first met, early in my career. Russ was a slender fit man with the posture of a sergeant in the army; he was a retired hospital administrator. His wife Marge was the supportive wife who stayed home and raised the children, like most women did in the 1950 and '60s. Upon retirement they moved to Florida and settled in. New habits were established while old ones became more ingrained and fixed. Marge was extremely proud of her German heritage and the stubbornness that went along with it. Marge and Russ came in to my office for their visits separately, keeping their medical problems private. Russ was proud of his great health and whenever I pointed out something that was awry, he was quick to address the problem. When he developed prostate cancer he had it attended to in a very efficient manner. Over the past year, he developed Parkinson's disease but declined medication thinking that he could work on his posture and make it go away. He showed a stubborn streak that reminded me of his wife.

Marge had rheumatoid arthritis and either did not tolerate medication or (more frequently) refused treatment, and as a result became more debilitated and disabled as time went by.

Every two years Russ would trade in his low-mileage Cadillac for a new one and each time I would wonder about his driving abilities or how the heck he got his wife in and out of the car to go to different restaurants each night for dinner.

Over the years I became very familiar with their routine and was lulled into a sense of false security that they were OK. That's why I was surprised when, one day, Russ came to the office after a motor vehicle accident. He claimed it was his fault, he did not see the light change. I snapped to attention, realizing that this man should not be driving. But he refused to consider relinquishing this freedom. Due to the damage from the accident he needed to trade for a new car and got a fire engine red Caddie. Hoping to prevent another accident (and commission for the Cadillac salesman), I started to gently advise consideration for a move to a facility where meals would be provided and he would no longer have to drive. He politely declined. I asked about his family; his son lived within an hour of their house but he told me, "They have busy lives," and he and Marge did not want to get them involved.

It was at this juncture that I recommend that they hire a Geriatric care manager. Russ showed polite interest when he inquired, "What is a geriatric care manger and what could they do for me?"

I took a deep breath as I knew getting Russ and Marge to buy into the concept would be a challenge. I explained that "geriatric care management (GCM) is the process of planning and coordinating care for aging adults like you and Marge who have physical and/or mental impairments to help meet their long term needs and, improve their quality of life and maintain their independence as long as possible. They work with patients and family (if desired) to develop and implement a plan using various social and health care services." Russ wrinkled his forehead indicating to me his skepticism but I ignored his gesture. I continued, "I have worked with many geriatric care managers over the years, they are all well trained and have experience in health and psychology, human development, family dynamics. They use public and private resources, and they know how to get funding when needed. In other words, they are advocates for their clients throughout the continuum of care. They work with all types of patient, especially with patients who suffer from dementia, frailty, and other chronic diseases."

I handed him a brochure, and I reviewed the various services that he and Marge could benefit. It included the following:

- Conducting care-planning assessments to identify needs, problems and eligibility for assistance
- Screening, arranging, and monitoring in-home help and other services
- Reviewing financial, legal, or medical issues
- Offering referrals to specialists to avoid future problems and to conserve assets
- Providing crisis intervention
- Acting as a liaison to families at a distance
- Making sure things are going well and alerting families of problems
- Assisting with moving their clients to or from a retirement complex, assisted living facility, rehabilitation facility or nursing home
- Providing client and family education and advocacy
- Offering counseling and support.

As our visit ended, Russ had acted as though he had never turned his hearing aide on for our visit. I hate that river "De-Nile".

As the months went by, Marge and Russ became more frail. They eventually faced reality and moved to a retirement community but by this time it was really too late for them to enjoy all the activities it had to offer. Marge developed a gastrointestinal infection with nausea and severe diarrhea. Russ was too weak and frail to get her out of bed, and she refused to go to the hospital until 10 days into the illness. By then, she was near death, extremely dehydrated and with a urinary tract infection. When she finally arrived in the hospital emergency room, my skills and modern medicine were able to bring her back from the brink but that's when things went from bad to worse.

I sent her to the rehabilitation facility located on the campus of the retirement community in which they lived, but she was not cooperative with the efforts of the rehab staff and made little progress. She was unable to provide her own self-care and her husband was too frail to provide it. Yet they both insisted they could get by. The staff made a home visit and determined that it was not safe for her to return to their house. When I asked about their children, to help with any transition, Russ said, "Oh, we don't have any contact with them anymore." *What a disaster*, I thought. How was I going to get them to arrive at a rational decision? My duty was to alert adult protective services if they went home under these circumstances. I offered options but they would not agree to help in the home. They dug in their heels; the answer was no. I guess this was their modus operandi when they were faced with a choice they did not like. They figured if they stared me down, eventually the staff and I would blink and they would get their way— the way they always had. Marge even suggested that all that could happen was that she would end up back in the hospital if she fell or if Russ could not get her out of bed. I told them I had far too much pride in my work to see that happen. Besides, she had already consumed more than $100,000 in medical care and so far there was little to show for it.

We went back and forth each week with these discussions. One day I would hear she would go home with 24-hour home health care, then hours later I would learn they changed their minds and she would stay in the nursing home for long term care. Another trip down that famous river in Egypt, De-Nile. What it is about people being so hung up about getting their own way, trying to be independent even when it's detrimental to their wellbeing?

My reminiscing ended as I arrived at my destination, where my family was gathering to celebrate Mom's birthday. She had chosen to have a small family dinner at her favorite restaurant, Runyons.

As we arrived, we sat down at a large round table, and awaited the other guests. First to arrive were my two 89 year old aunts (they had a habit of arriving promptly). Aunt Jeanette had Alzheimer's disease and despite being told about dinner 5 times that day she had already eaten her dinner. "I just was hungry and I forgot about dinner," she apologized. Aunt Eleanor was great, a real sharp mind but deaf as a doorknob. Next to arrive was my brother, Lewis, with his 16 year old daughter, Danni, and his girlfriend, Lisa.

There was a lot of commotion at the table as we ordered drinks. As we settled in, I listened to Lisa talk about her 70 year old mother, Ruth. I had met Ruth once or twice before but had not really gotten to know her at all. Through the clamor and noise I heard how Ruth, widowed for just one year, had met a man. Lisa spoke to Ruth regularly and while happy about the blossoming relationship, she did not want to know the details of a sexual relationship between her 70 year old mother and 77 year old widower. "It's awkward and embarrassing to discuss this with my mother. Too much information and salacious details," exclaimed Lisa.

I listened with interest and I was not surprised that the daughter, Lisa, knew very little about what is going on. The fact is that I knew *exactly* what is going on. This is the type of story I had heard over and over again from my patients for the past 30 years. Older adults are desperate to be heard and understood. They appreciate me as a non-judgmental listener, someone who has heard the story before, who can validate their feeling and give sage advice. I am sure that this is one of the reasons I enjoy taking care of older adults. These people romance each other without the games young people play. Then, if things seem right, they become intimate.

The comfort level to which I am referring doesn't start with a first visit. It takes time, often years. As patients begin to respect and trust me, and get to know me, a special bond develops. To me, getting below the surface with my patients is another gratifying part of my job. Clearly my patients want to get to know the person to whom they entrust their lives, but I learn much about myself as I let them in. Most patients want to know that I am human like them; they want to know that I have children like they do. They enjoy hearing that my children, like theirs, have their successes and failures alike. So these office visits often run a bit longer and I fall behind in my schedule. However this sets the tone so when the need arises for them to ask a very intimate question they know me not just as a doctor but as a person and feel they can trust I will understand the sensitivity of the moment and be able to give them the guidance they seek. Whether the subject is related to the end of life or the beginning of a new relationship, I will have insight because I understand them well enough to provide them with the direction they need to face their fears or uncertainty.

Peggy is a good example. I have been taking care of her for the past 10 years and her precious husband, Tony, for five years before she became a patient. She wanted to make sure she could relate to me. She loved Tony and was a devoted wife. Her world revolved around him. Tony had prostate cancer; he had been treated by an expert, the department chair at the local medical school. He had received cutting edge therapy at the time and had lived beyond what might have been his predicted life expectancy. Unfortunately, the treatment he received left him impotent. When I met them both for the first time we discussed this sensitive issue and I learned that they had a great marriage, loved each other very much and sex (or the lack thereof) was not an issue at all. I treated Tony for multiple medical problems in an era before Viagra had been discovered and the topic of sex was not discussed. Advanced prostate cancer is frequently treated with medication that counteracts the effects of testosterone and therefore libido is usually absent. This type of treatment has negative effects in many different areas of the body including the ability to form bones. Tony developed osteoporosis and suffered the painful effects of spinal fractures. On one such occasion he was sent to the hospital to have a procedure to put cement in the fractured bone to bolster it, promote healing and to reduce his pain. During the procedure he suffered a complication and died. In the weeks after Tony's death Peggy visited me with her daughter. She asked for clarification of the events. "Doctor, what happened? Why did Tony die? Did Tony make a mistake by choosing to have this procedure?" she inquired. I explained what had happened during his procedure and that it was "just his time." "Peggy, Tony always made good decisions about his health, and had he not been as attentive as he was he would have died long ago," I responded. My remarks went a long way toward settling her mind and she thanked me for the good care I had always given Tony. She added, "Tony always told me how much he appreciated your kindness and attentiveness in answering all his questions and what you had done for him while he was alive. He really trusted you, Dr. Bernstein."

During the next few months I saw Peggy in the office and counseled her through her grieving process. I consider it an honor to help my patients through this process, especially if they do not have the opportunity to interact with a member of the clergy.

"It usually takes about a year to pass all of the milestones of a life before the grief process comes to an end. There will be the first Christmas, first birthday and first anniversary without him, and then there will be a Thanksgiving," I explain.

Toward the end of the first year after a spouse's death I frequently ask if there is any interest in becoming involved in a relationship again. This usually catches the patient off-guard, but then I often hear, "I am not really interested in that, Doctor." My favorite line came many years ago from a patient named Frieda. When I asked the question and she responded with, "Hell no, Doc, to cook, clean and pick up after another man again, that would be ridiculous." When I asked Peggy, she just said, "Tony was one of a kind and could never be replaced. I am not looking". It was this development in our relationship that enabled Peggy to trust that she could speak about anything with me.

Over the ensuing years Peggy would come to the office for routine monitoring of her blood pressure and to flirt with me. I would say, "Peggy you are so charming, you make me blush." She was on what I call "cruise control." The medication I had chosen had always worked well and she would use the extra time we had together to spar about one thing or another. About eight years after her husband's death, Peggy was in my office for one of those easy visits when she told me that a man had expressed interest in her. It was her old boss. He lived in Ohio and would be spending some of the winter near her in Florida. She informed me that they were just old friends and they would probably go out to dinner once or twice while he was in town. With a tilt of my head and a raise of an eyebrow, I wondered out loud if she thought he had other interests. She told me, "It's too bad if he did because I have no desire to become involved with a man at this time."

I did not see Peggy for another three months, until she returned in the late spring. She told me that the visit with her "old friend" went well and she was planning to take a trip to visit him in the upcoming months of the summer. Now I raised both eyebrows and inquired, "What has provoked your change in attitude?" I could see her soften a little as she told me, "I had a very nice time with this man and he was a perfect gentleman." She continued, "I will be staying at his home in the guest bedroom." I nodded my head and asked, "What do you expect of this trip?" She naively exclaimed, "That we will continue to spend time together and do some traveling." She was taken aback when I asked, "When do you intend to sleep with this man?" She said, "Come on, Dr. Bernstein, that is not what he is interested in. He is my former boss and just wants to be friends with me." I laughed out loud; she was surprised but neither embarrassed nor offended, asking, "What's so funny?"

I waited to respond; the silence was deafening. I explained, "Peggy, I have listened to similar stories many times over the years; the naive woman goes to visit the man. They are bound to become physical sooner rather than later." She told me, "This idea is preposterous!"

She was "a good Catholic girl." It would never happen! "Besides," she exclaimed, "I would have to be married before I would sleep with him." She went on to tell me how ridiculous sleeping with this man would be. You see, Peggy was a virgin when she married Tony and he was the only man she had ever slept with. Plus, because of his condition, they had not had sex in 16 years. Before she left my office, I suggested that she be open-minded to the possibility that, if a relationship were to develop, what she might expect and what she needed to consider. My parting remarks pertained to the fact that this man was probably very interested in her and had a strong interest in sleeping with her—I told her I suspected it would be sooner rather than later.

Peggy came to see me in the fall for her routine blood pressure visit. Before I had a chance to ask about her summer trip, she blurted out my five favorite words, "Dr. Bernstein, you were right." Her eyes lit up and she smiled broadly.

"Tell me what happened?" There was no blushing as she started to tell me how this man romanced her. "Details, details," I requested. I hardly had to ask. She was very forthright and told me many of the details of how wonderful her experiences were—the man was gentle and there was never a second of embarrassment with him. I even asked what went through her mind when she disrobed to reveal her 75 year old body. "It was as natural as anything else I had ever done," she said. At the end of our discussion she added, "I cannot thank you enough for bringing up this delicate subject and preparing me for my adventure."

What Ruth and Peggy demonstrate and many of my other patients reinforce during their visits is their desire for closeness and intimacy for as long as they live. It seems apparent to me that both men and women derive pleasure out of intimacy or a close relationship. Generally, men are more sexual while women appear to thrive on the relationship. Those who are fortunate to find the middle ground between sexuality and a close relationship can find exciting new experiences in later life.

The stories in this chapter would lead one to wonder if there are common themes of aging... the stories demonstrate the vast spectrum of issues and emotions that aging adults live through. The people in these stories show a clear desire to maintain a happy and independent life without intrusion from children or authority figures. There is juxtaposition however between the weakening grip on personal choices and the development of a new and exciting beginning. The goal is always the same: a life that is as healthy and independent as possible with the potential for fulfillment.

After years of observing patient's lives, I have seen patterns that would have developed early in life or in a relationship. There are those who get stuck in "their ways" and become more of what they were: inflexible. There are others with more positive attitudes who demonstrate greater flexibility, who are able to adapt more readily to what is dealt to them and can "go with the flow."

Notes on Living Longer

- "As people get older, they become more of what they always were." As we age we tend to get more set in our ways, more resistant to change and become less flexible in our daily routines and approach to life.
- As we age, we strive to be as independent as possible, to maintain a status quo while risking adverse consequences in favor of a safer and more restrictive environment.
- Intimacy, love and companionship are natural desires/needs in life no matter how long we live. How we approach new relationships later in life may challenge us, may make us uncomfortable or giddy and make us think. These natural desires can challenge our previously

held belief system, resulting in greater fulfillment of life.

- Be cognizant of your behavior as you age. Are you more of what you were, more set in our ways? Consider adaptations.
- Be willing to compromise and make changes in your level of independence in order to enhance your well-being and reduce risk for injury and other adverse outcomes.
- Trust your instincts to be drawn to new relationships, love and intimacy.
- Work toward maintaining strong family relationships as they can be important later in life.

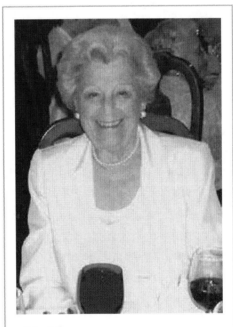

My Mother, the philosopher

Resources:

Helpguide.org, *Better Senior Sex: Tips for Enjoying a Healthy Sex Life as You Age*, retrieved November 3, 2011 from http://www.helpguide.org/elder/sexuality_aging.htm

Staff, Mayo Clinic(2011) *Sexual health and aging: Keep the passion alive;* Retrieved April 12, 2012 from http://www.mayoclinic.com/health/sexual-health/HA00035

Wild, Carleen (2010) *Intimacy and Aging*, Retrieved November 2011, from http://www.nbc15.com/news/headlines/93704099.html

Center on Aging Studies at the University of Missouri-Kansas City (UMKC), University of Missouri Outreach and Extension Successful Aging; *Sexuality/Intimacy/ Companionship/Family*

Retrieved November 2011 from http://cas.umkc.edu/casww/SA/sex.htm#INTERNET%20REFERENCES

National Association of Geriatric Care Manager, www.caremanager.org

Chapter 7

Environment

If I'd known how old I was going to be I'd have taken better care of myself.
– **Adolph Zukor**

To lengthen thy life, lessen thy meals.
– **Benjamin Franklin**

M any years ago while having lunch at a local restaurant with my parents, a short elderly woman approached and greeted my mother. After exchanging a few pleasantries, my mother introduced me to her friend Mildred. She seemed to be a pleasant woman and looked well. I was taken by the rather peculiar sweater she was wearing: it had pictures of her grandchildren sewn into a series of square sections that ran across the front of the blue cardigan.

"Mom," I inquired after Mildred had left, "what's up with that lady with the sweater?"

Mom responded, "Would you believe that woman is 90 years old, is in excellent health, and she has practiced yoga every day for the last 40 years?"

I marveled at how healthy this woman looked at age 90, how upright her posture was, and the confidence with which she walked. Obviously, Mildred knew how to adapt to her environment.

How *does* environment play a role in how we live our lives? Environment—the world around us, how we interact, and what we do within the environment in which we live—plays a major role in how we maintain our health. The life-choices people make and how they practice healthy lifestyles are key, and are the personal attributes to a longer, happier and more fulfilling life. Keep in mind, these are *choices*; along with a good attitude, good health is the outcome.

In preparing this chapter, I was challenged to select among the many patients in my practice who illustrate how to favorably interact with the environment. Generally, people who practice healthy lifestyles become ill infrequently and therefore do not see a physician very often, in contrast to my "frequent fliers." In addition, these healthy individuals make a routine health-maintenance visit only every one to two years. In a 25 year career, I might get to see a patient like this just 10 to 15 times in my interaction in their 80 to 90 year lifespan. The point is this: people who lead healthy lifestyles really don't get sick very often and don't have much opportunity to stand out like the patients who interact poorly with their environment.

Michael, a patient of mine, stands as an example of a person making poor lifestyle choices. He is a 53 year old man I see about every 3 months—if he remembers his appointments. I have been his physician for at least a dozen years and when he comes to my office I attempt to provide guidance. I don't consider that I am able to provide good care though when he does not adhere to my suggestions to improve his lifestyle. He is married to a woman he can no longer tolerate; it's a loveless marriage. He is obese, eats very poorly, and shows no motivation to make healthier choices. Over the last six years, I have diagnosed him with high blood pressure, diabetes, and high cholesterol. He has had emergency visits to the hospital on at least three occasions for heart catheterization and had stents placed in the arteries that supply blood to his heart. Despite all this, he has demonstrated a clear inability or unwillingness to change his diet, lose weight or exercise. Since I informed him that he had diabetes, he has not tested his blood sugars anywhere near the frequency I recommended and has declined going to a dietician or for diabetic education. He has even admitted to me that he has some emotional problems leading to depression but has refused to discuss these issues with a mental health professional. Despite his refusal to interact with his environment in an intelligent fashion, what I don't understand is how he has not died yet. While he stands out in my practice, he is not alone in our society in neglecting how he interacts with his environment.

Scientific literature on diet, exercise, and other health practices is considerable but often marred by small sample sizes. Large population studies are not common due to the enormous challenges associated with cost, the need for large number of subjects, and the duration of follow-up needed. Review of this data is beyond the scope of this book. I will, however, focus on those attributes that I have noted which seem to provide the greatest influence on living longer and healthier lives.

Lawrence J. Appel reports that "in The Nurses' Health Study *(Circulation. 2008)*, a large prospective, observational study of 72,113 female nurses who were free of coronary artery disease, stroke, diabetes and cancer were followed over an 18 year period of time. Two diet patterns were observed. One pattern (called *prudent)* was defined by the high consumption of vegetables, fruit, legumes, fish, poultry and whole grains. The other group was called (*Western),* typical of an American diet that included a high consumption of red meat, processed meat, refined grains, French fries, sweets and desserts. In comparing the two groups there was a considerable difference (20% to 30%) in total mortality, cardiovascular mortality, and non-cardiovascular mortality. It was noted that there was no difference in cancer mortality rates in the two groups. It is worth pointing out that throughout the world there are other diets that have fared well with regard to longevity when studied under similar circumstances. The traditional Okinawan diet (*Asia Pac J Clin Nutr*) provides more than 90% of calories from carbohydrates (predominantly vegetables), whereas the Mediterranean diet provides less than 40% of its calories from fat, mostly monounsaturated and polyunsaturated fat. Each of these diets, along with diets with low caloric intake, has been associated with longer life expectancies."

I enjoy seeing my older patients who have interacted in a healthy way with their environment. One such patient I've cared for greater than 25 years is Georgette. I met her when she was 60, married, and very active. She would talk to me about her world travels and her healthy lifestyle. She told me how much she enjoyed being active including taking dance, stretching, and yoga several times a week. (She was one of the inspirations that got me started practicing yoga myself.) To this day, I recall her words and her thick New York accent as she said, "Doctor, yoga is a non-judgmental activity. No one will judge you in class based on how much you stretch and what you do." Every time I go to yoga class, I recall her words.

Georgette has rarely been ill; I have treated her when she developed minor problems associated with menopause and an underactive thyroid. These were easily treated, and she has been very adherent with her medication. She became widowed after I had known her for five years and continued an active lifestyle. She would travel across the country to visit friends and family or fly off to Europe or Asia or Antarctica when she could find someone to travel with. When not traveling, she would go to her exercise classes four or five times a week. Several other patients in my practice knew her from these classes but had no idea of her age. She ate a very simple healthy diet. She was careful not to expose herself to undo health risks. She did not smoke, her alcohol consumption was minimal, and she was very careful not to involve herself in any risky behaviors. We would talk about risky behaviors from time to time because I thought it was important to warn my patients about certain dangers I had observed over the years: having an accident while working on a roof, or falling off a ladder or stepstool while changing a light bulb can have devastating consequences and ruin what had been a peaceful and happy life. I've always felt that it was very important for me to share my concerns about these risks with my patients. In my older patient population there have been very few taking risks such as skydiving or motorcycle riding and none of my patients in this age group have ever performed in a rodeo after the age of 60. I consider those wise choices.

Georgette had other healthy habits. Her diet was mostly vegetarian. She meditated almost every day. She interacted with people in her classes, especially those younger than she. In her early 80s, she told me she was having problems with her memory and anxiety. She tried her best to use meditation to help with this but when it was not effective enough, she did accept my recommendation to take medication, which was quite effective for the anxiety. With regard to her memory, we found that her continuation of exercise and remaining active allowed her to function quite well without the need for medication. It was important for her to maintain her independence although her children frequently offered to help when needed.

Since stress due to work, finances, and the rigors of nurturing a family has become such a common problem in our society, it is not surprising to see so many people looking for alternative methods of relaxation. Yoga, which was developed in India more than 4000 years ago is considered a mind-body type of complementary and alternative medicine practice (but it does not require a prescription). By stretching and toning muscles, flexing the spine and focusing the mind inward, Yoga brings together physical and mental disciplines to achieve peacefulness of body and mind, leading to help with relaxation, reduction in anxiety and management of stress. Chronic stress has been shown to have a negative effect on many systems in the human body most notably the cardiovascular system. Yoga, along with meditation, has been shown to reduce heart rate and blood pressure and as a result has been incorporated into many cardiac rehabilitation programs. Yoga has been credited with helping people lose weight, develop an enhanced feeling of well-being, and calming the mind. It is likely that the practice of Yoga and meditation has an effect on neurotransmitters in the brain that lead to these effects. Yoga can lead to a more toned and fit appearance, and improve movement and balance as we age. Recall my mother's 90-year old friend Mildred from earlier in this chapter.

Bruce came to me as a new patient when he was 60. He had moved to Florida from Michigan, where he had worked in the automobile industry as a tool and die maker. This was not a very prestigious job but he was proud of it and felt he retired with a decent pension. Bruce believed in keeping active and living in a community that offered a full range of activities including a fitness center. He would use the treadmill or swim almost every day, and he played in a senior softball league two times a week. He was attentive to his diet as well. I monitored his cholesterol, which for the most part was well controlled. Despite his diligent efforts of diet, exercise, and stress reduction, one day he developed tightness in his chest. I initiated a routine work up for chest pain that lead to a heart catheterization. This test revealed a blockage in one of his coronary arteries. A stent was inserted into his right coronary artery and for the next 20 years he had no further chest tightness. Despite his excellent diet, I convinced him that medication could be effective in addition to his diet in helping prevent another event. With some prodding and cajoling he agreed, and he was able to continue to play in his senior softball league at least to the age of 86. Bruce was very proud of the fact that he never smoked cigarettes, always ate a healthy diet, and exercised six days a week. He told me that his parents had heart disease and they died in their mid-60s and how grateful that, in his mid-80s, he had already lived well beyond that.

Some of the men with whom he played softball were younger than he—others were as much as 10 years older. He enjoyed the camaraderie with all of them and it provided an additional positive feature in his environment. It's interesting to note that his meals at home with his wife were very healthy yet his wife was nowhere near as active as he was. Bruce controlled his own environment by remaining active, eating right, and interacting with other like-minded individuals. Particularly because he considered himself a 'macho' male, I periodically reminded him of the dangers associated with risky environmental behaviors. Much like I had with Georgette, I described "risky environment behaviors" as the dangers of ladders, step stools, and poor judgment when driving (rush hour, night driving, and making left turns). We were in agreement with the driving restrictions. Additionally, it was evident that playing softball into his 80s did present some risks. He did suffer with severe arthritis of his hip, possibility related to his sporting activities, and eventually required a hip replacement. Six months after the hip replacement, however, he was back playing softball. He then suffered from shoulder problems, had arthroscopic surgery, and worked very hard at rehabilitation in the off-season so he didn't miss a game when the new season began.

Our entire society has become far too sedentary for a multitude of reasons. In the past half century we have seen a meteoric rise in obesity, diabetes and cardiovascular diseases. Studies have shown that individuals of all ages can improve quality of life and reduce the risk of developing coronary heart disease, hypertension, type 2 diabetes mellitus, and some cancers by participating in moderate physical activity and exercise. Regular exercise programs promote improved musculoskeletal function and enhance your mental well-being, too.

Since cardiovascular disease is the leading cause of death among both sexes in the U.S., exercise has been studied as a modifier of that risk. Moderate exercise of *as little as* 30 minutes a day has been shown to reduce risk of cardiac events. This same amount of physical activity has been shown to improve insulin sensitivity in diabetics and to reduce blood pressure in hypertensive patients.

Kravitz (2007) reports that "muscle mass, strength, power and endurance have been shown to decrease with age but it has been suggested that this is largely due to a decrease in physical activity and not necessarily age alone. There is a linear relationship with loss of muscle strength and loss of independence, contributing to falls, fractures and admissions to nursing homes. Sarcopenia is the age-related loss of muscle mass and strength. It has been noted that starting at age 50, the typical adult will lose one to two percent of muscle mass per year (Marcell 2003). This can be mitigated by regular exercise and strength training. The improvement in musculoskeletal health allows elderly individuals to perform activities of daily living more effectively and with less effort. Guidelines have been established for resistance training for sarcopenia prevention (ACSM 2006)."

In my practice I see many patients with nervous system diseases: depression, anxiety, insomnia, and dementia. The antidepressant and antianxiety action is one of the most commonly accepted benefits of exercise. It has been shown that 25 to 60 minutes of aerobic exercise improves mood and decreases negative feelings. The further effects often improve sleep patterns. Studies have shown that increased physical activity has resulted in significantly favorable improvement in patients with Alzheimer's disease as well.

My mother's friend Mildred and my patients Bruce and Georgette are excellent examples of people who control their own environment rather than having it control them. They have incorporated scientifically proven activities and behaviors into their lives for positive results. In addition, Bruce and Georgette follow recommendations from their doctor to compliment the positive things they do. Of the five attributes of GRACE, interacting with our environment might be the one we have the most control over. I urge my patients and others who want to live long and productive lives to adjust unhealthy habits to some of the more favorable ones addressed in this chapter. I hope their stories will inspire you to do the same.

Notes on living longer:

- There is a plethora of literature supporting the benefits of leading a healthy lifestyle.
- Seeking medical attention to assist in the controlling of known risk factors like high blood pressure and high cholesterol have significant and documented benefits.
- Having periodic health maintenance examinations to discuss additional risk can be extremely beneficial in promoting longevity and quality of life.

- Avoiding unhealthy practices like smoking, driving when impaired, and participating in other hazardous activities such as climbing on ladders and roofs have unseen benefits.
- Become educated about healthy lifestyles choices at an early age to gain the lifelong benefits.
- Consult with your physician when you have questions about practices that can lead to a longer and happier life.

Resources and Links:

National Institute on Aging (NIA)(2011)*Exercise & Physical Activity: Your Everyday Guide from the National Institute on Aging*. Retrieved November 6, 2011 from http://www.nia.nih.gov/health/publication/exercise-physical-activity-your-everyday-guide-national-institute-aging-1

Exercise for Seniors: MedlinePlus http://www.nlm.nih.gov/medlineplus/exerciseforseniors.html

Harvard Health Publications; Harvard Medical School http://www.health.harvard.edu/topic/aging

Park, Alice (2010) *Studies Link Exercise in Older Adults to Healthier Aging* Retrieved November 6, 2011 from www.time.com/time/health/article/0,8599,1956619,00.html

Goel, Arun (2006) *Reverse Aging Through Yoga – Part I & II,* Retrieved January 20, 2012 from ***http://www.healthandyoga.com***

Lucas, Marsha *Rewire Your Brain for Love: Creating Vibrant Relationships Using the Science of Mindfulness* (Hay House, 2012)

Staff, Mayo Clinic (2010) _Yoga:Tap in to the Many Health Benefits._ Retrieved November 06, 2011from http://www.mayoclinic.com/health/yoga/CM00004

Francina, Suza (2007) _Yoga Solutions for Healthy Aging_. Retrieved November 16, 2011| from ELDR.com, www.eldr.com/article/fitness/yoga-solutions-healthy-aging

Alzheimer's Association, _Brain Health_, Retrieved November 16, 2011from Alz.org/We Can Help, **http://www.alz.org/we_can_help_brain_health_maintain_your_brain.asp**

Healthy Brain Initiative, A National Public Health Road Map to Maintaining Cognitive Health. Retrieved August 30, 2012 from the Alzheimer's Association http://www.alz.org/national/documents/report_healthybraininitiative.pdf

Harford County Maryland, Dept of Community Services, Office on Aging (2007) _Home Safety Check-List_ Retrieved November 16, 2011 from www.harfordcountymd.gov/services/aging/HomeSafety.html

NIH: National Institute on Aging (2010) Home Safety for People with Alzheimer's Disease, Retrieved November 16, 2011 from http://www.nia.nih.gov/alzheimers/publication/home-safety-people-alzheimers-disease

Texas AgriLife Extension Service,Family and Consumer Sciences. _Aging, elder care, safety, health and aging, senior medications._ Retrieved November 16, 2011 from AgriLife.org http://fcs.tamu.edu/families/aging/index.php

Safeaging.org, Safe Aging; _Falls Prevention; Senior Safety; Injury Prevention._ Retrieved November 16, 2011 from www.safeaging.org

Chapter 8

Begin With the End in Mind

Begin with the end in mind is based on the principle that all is created twice. There is a mental or first creation, and a physical or second creation to all things.

– Stephen Covey

In my practice of medicine, an essential component of my approach with each patient is based on a Stephen Covey teaching: *Begin with the end in mind*. It is also a strategy I use on the golf course, but more about that later. As a physician who works with late middle-age to advanced old-age individuals—the standard profile being multiple coexisting and complex medical problems—I've learned that taking a fast-forward look at the most realistic ending is the best way to develop an optimal treatment plan. While it sounds dramatic, the process is slow and hardly ever gets anyone's attention. A lot like the game of golf.

On the golf course, I've learned to play each hole backwards in my mind before I take the first swing. It works like this: the first hole at the course I play in Florida is a 500 yard par five. My goal is to get the ball into the hole in five strokes, which means swing number four has to land the ball on the green, and close enough to the hole for me to sink a putt (that would have to be within two feet because putting has never been my strong suit.) This means my third shot has to land somewhere near enough to the green for me to hit a chip shot that will drop the ball within the two foot range I need to sink the putt. In order for me to get to that point, I need to launch my second shot about 130 yards from the green. That means I need a tee shot of 200 yards and the ball needs to land somewhere in the middle of the fairway. While this may sound straightforward, I've neglected to mention that the golf course designer placed hazards and obstacles along the way. There is a creek running along the entire left side of the hole (yes, there are alligators in that creek); there are trees lining the entire right side of the fairway; and the green is surrounded by five enormous sand traps. Similar to the pitfalls of living in a body with some years on it.

When I first met Mel, it was 1988, a time before cardiac stents were widely used and definitely before stents for other blood vessels had been invented. Were he a patient of mine today, his treatment and prognosis would have been quite different. He was new to my practice and was a nervous, compulsive 86 year old. He was, I later learned, a retired engineer.

Mel was my last patient of the day. It was three thirty and I was beginning to tire as my workday had started at four that morning when I'd been awakened by a call from a hospital nurse reporting an abnormal lab result. Mel arrived at my office accompanied by his wife. He was dressed casually in dark slacks and a faded blue button-down short-sleeve shirt, with several mechanical pencils stuck in the breast pocket. He looked his age, with thin grey hair and a slow gait. His expression suggested concern and anxiety. His wife, Violet, was neat, demure and seemingly attentive to all of his needs. Clearly, he was the "pack leader" and she followed along, supportive and submissive. If she *did* disagree with something he said, she showed no signs of disapproval.

At his side, Mel had a leather attaché case in which he carried several neatly organized file folders. Each folder was part of a well-organized system, with pockets for blood tests, x-rays results, consultation reports, and prescriptions. He pulled out a red folder.

"Good afternoon, Mr. Smith. It's nice to meet you," I said as I escorted the couple into my consultation room.

"Nice to meet you, Dr. Bernstein. My name is Mel and this is my wife, Violet." He sat down in a chair across from my desk and glanced out the window. "What a peaceful view you have here," he said.

I have always been fond of the view from my consultation room. It is beautiful and serene, with tall cypress trees anchored in marsh, offering glimpses of local Florida wildlife. That scene always made it hard to believe we are in an office building only 200 yards from one of the busiest roads in the state of Florida.

"How may help you, Mr. Smith? Or shall I call you Mel?"

"Please, call me Mel." He opened his red folder. "My previous physician didn't seem to have the time or interest in me anymore so I am switching physicians."

I leaned forward to show interest. He fumbled with the folder for a few seconds before I said, "Please, Mel, put your folder aside and just tell me how you're feeling today." He seemed relieved that I had expressed an interest in understanding exactly how he felt.

"I'm just really tired, Doc, and nobody takes me seriously. I have a cardiologist who just prescribes medications for my angina, I have a gastroenterologist who gives me medication for my heartburn, I went to my orthopedist who gave me arthritis pills. But no one seems to have gotten to the bottom of why I'm so tired all the time."

It was clear he was very concerned about his health. I wanted to put him at ease and at the same time get to know him better. "Mel, I would really first just like to know more about you. I see that you came with your wife today; tell me, how long have you been married?"

Mel began to relax as he talked, and I learned he had been married for 60 years and had three children. He had been a civil engineer for most of his career and had owned his own business. He and his wife enjoyed traveling, and were active socially. He spoke proudly of his grandchildren.

This was my first encounter with an engineer as a patient. In fact, I didn't know any engineers in life outside my practice. Since my acquaintance with Mel, however, I've had several other patients who were retired engineers and I have found them all to be similarly challenging; they are inquisitive by nature (and, no doubt, by training) and come with a litany of questions to which they want definitive answers. I remember one time telling an engineer patient that his cholesterol had dropped, from 205 to 197. He stopped talking for a moment, performing the calculation in his head, and told me those numbers represented a 4-percent reduction, a figure he found to be statistically significant. I had to remind him that the small change represented only the standard daily variation in his body or an acceptable variability within the lab analyzer.

Mel continued talking and I learned that he had coronary artery disease, well-controlled with medication, and his angina attacks were infrequent. We agreed that my responsibility would be to help him manage his complex medical problems, which included not only his coronary artery disease but also hypertension, high cholesterol, and an underactive thyroid gland. After about 30 minutes discussing his medical history, my nurse took him into my exam room. While Mel was left to undress and put on an examination gown, I stayed behind and reviewed the thick folder of his medical records now on my desk. I took my time, carefully reading page after page of reports from Mel's blood tests, EKGs, and X-rays from his cardiologist. Later, photocopies would be made for my own file.

I found Mel sitting quietly on my exam table, stripped to his underwear. I performed a thorough exam, focusing my attention on his neck and thyroid gland, his heart and lungs, his abdomen, and his mental status. Afterward, he and his wife rejoined me in my consultation room.

"What did you find, Doc?" was Mel's first questions.

"Well, Mel, I would like more time to review your records and run some routine blood tests, but you seem to be doing quite well. Your blood pressure is still on the high side and I will increase one of your medications today but other than that things look really good for a man your age." I handed him some written instructions and asked him to schedule an appointment to return in two weeks.

Over the next few months we had several visits together. I would adjust his blood pressure medicines and answer his latest round of questions: "How does that blood pressure medicine work?" "How come you use such a low dose of Procardia [30mg] and such a high dose of Metoprolol [200 mg]?" "Why am I on such a low dose of Synthroid when I am always so tired?" I enjoyed these conversations, and with each visit we established greater rapport.

He continued to complain of fatigue. When my explanations did not satisfy his inquisitive engineering mind, he decided finally to seek the opinion of an endocrinologist. I could not blame the man; he had a high level of curiosity and obsessivness. He found an excellent physician to do the evaluation and one of the considerations (although quite unlikely) was that the fatigue could have been caused by a problem in the adrenal gland. A far-fetched idea, considering that the patient had lived 86 years before developing this problem, *and* he had several more compelling reasons to have fatigue: In addition to his age, his heart disease, his high blood pressure and several of the medicines he was taking were far more likely culprits. In any event, the endocrinologist ordered a CT scan *; no adrenal abnormality was detected. There was, however, a 7.5 cm abdominal aortic aneurysm* (also called a "triple A") that the scan revealed and the patient was promptly sent back to me by the endocrinologist so that I could decide what to do about it.

The aorta is the main blood vessel that carries blood away from the heart to the rest of the body. An aneurysm is an abnormal enlargement in the wall of a blood vessel. An abdominal aortic aneurysm, therefore, is an abnormal enlargement of the lower part of the aorta as it extends through the abdominal area. The aorta is an elastic blood vessel, filled with blood that's under pressure as it is pumped from the heart.

Aneurysms can develop in weakened segments of the blood vessel wall, distending it like a balloon. When I describe aneurysms to my patients, I tell them it is like a bubble in a garden hose.

The major predisposing factors contributing to the development of an aneurysm are smoking, family history, congenital defects, injury, infection, and high blood pressure. Each year in the U.S., abdominal aortic aneurysms cause 15,000 deaths. The majority of these deaths are due to the sudden rupture of the aneurysm and rapid internal bleeding. Aneurysms can be diagnosed with a physical exam (by palpation), and by routine radiological tests such as X-rays, CT scans and MRI. Sometimes they are detected as what's called an "incidental finding" on one of these radiological tests. A study performed in the 1960's revealed that the risk of rupture was directly related to the size of the aneurysm—the larger the aneurysm, the greater the risk. This was the knowledge base available to me when I was treating Mel. The treatment at that time was to send these patients (who by nature of the condition were old), through a major abdominal operation to replace the dilated aortic, to prevent its rupture and the patient's certain death.

The endocrinologist had passed the hot potato to me. Now, with Mel's latest diagnosis, I was faced with several difficult tasks. The first was to explain the results of a test that I had neither ordered nor thought necessary. I have always found it difficult to put myself in the shoes (or brain) of another physician. The philosophy I follow in my practice comes from advice I was given by my chief resident when I was an intern: *"A test is only as good as the question you are asking."* In this situation, *I* had not asked the question. At least I had a copy of the consultation indicating the rationale for ordering the CT scan. Next, I had to figure out what to do with an 86 year old man with a fairly large AAA. Mel's aneurysm had a likelihood of rupturing sometime within the next two to three years and, if not operated on within this period of time, would likely lead to Mel's sudden death.

I thought the case through before discussing it with Mel. He had severe coronary artery disease and the standard of care at the time was to perform a coronary artery bypass (CABG) first and then do the repair of the AAA. In a man his age, his recovery from heart bypass—if all went well—would take 6 months before he was back on his feet and ready to have his AAA fixed. It would take him another 6 months to recover completely from the AAA repair. Assuming his life expectancy was 88, he would have spent one of the last two years of his life recovering from two major surgeries. It just did not seem to me to be a sensible idea to have the surgery.

We met again in my consultation room with the windows that overlooked the cypress trees. Mel had his red folder full of test results and on the other side the desk I had a manila file folder full of all his tests and lab reports. He initiated the conversation. "Dr. Bernstein, I would like to discuss the CT scan report and ask your advice about having it [AAA] cut out. Who is the best surgeon for the job? The doctor who ordered the CT scan told me very little and instructed me to discuss this whole situation with you." *Yes*, I thought to myself, *he certainly did!*

What made an already complex conversation more difficult was the fact that Mel was a man who lived in the "black and white" world of engineering—far from the nuanced art and science of medicine. I needed to be delicate, and gentle, while providing him with a great deal of information. Information that would, ultimately, tell him how he was likely to die.

I started the conversation. "Mel, I have had a chance to review your latest test result, the CT scan ordered by your endocrinologist. I have spent a lot of time considering how to manage your case, but before I begin, I would like to hear your thoughts,."

He responded, "Well, Doctor, I don't have much choice. I figure I have to have the aneurysm cut out or I am going to die. Are there any other options that you can think of?"

"Mel, this is how I see it," I remarked. "You are living a pretty content life and enjoy traveling and doing things around the house. You and your wife go out to dinner and visit family whenever you want. It is a real blessing at your age to be able to do these things. I suggest that you continue living your life just the way you are right now."

He was startled that I did not suggest an operation to repair his aortic aneurysm. "This is how I see it, Mel," I began again. "You have advanced coronary artery disease, so before the aneurysm can be repaired, you will have to have a heart bypass operation. It is likely to take six months for you to recover from that surgery before you would be well enough to undergo a repair of your aortic aneurysm. Assuming all goes well with the repair of your aneurysm, you will be recovering for an additional six months before you are *where you are today.* I figure you currently have a life expectancy of 2 years right now, so, if you proceed with surgery you will spend *one of the last two years of your life recovering from surgery.* It does not make sense to me."

Mel had been listening intently and nodded that he understood. "Doctor, you've made excellent points that I had not considered. I would like to go home and mull over your recommendation and see you again in a week or so. Would that be acceptable with you?"

"Sure," I said with an inward sense of relief, "that would be great. I look forward to discussing this again with you then."

A few weeks later Mel returned with his wife. We sat in my office to review his options again. "Doctor Bernstein, I have made up my mind," he started. "I heard everything you said to me at my last visit and I have done some calculations on my own and I agree with your appraisal. It would be too risky for me to undergo two such invasive operations at my age. Violet and I have talked this over at great length and she is very supportive of my decision. Next week we are planning on going to California to visit an old high school friend and then we will drive up the coast to Oregon to visit our children and grandchildren. We have put that trip off for a long time and I think now is the right time to go."

Over the next year Mel returned for follow up visits every three months. Although he was still obsessed about his blood pressure and cholesterol, he was more relaxed about it than that day he first walked into my office. At these visits we discussed other important issues as well. We talked about his finances, his life insurance, his Will, his Advance Directives and Living Will. He made sure to get each in order and he discussed them with Violet and his children. Seeing to these matters gave him a sense of relief, he told me. At one of our sessions, he told me about a recent trip to Niagara Falls, where he and his wife had honeymooned many years earlier, and to his 60th college reunion. He had become comfortable and relaxed with his decision, and went about living.

Nearly three years after we first met, I received a call from my hospital's emergency room. Mel has suffered chest pains at home that lasted about 10 minutes before he collapsed. He was brought to the ER but upon his arrival he had no pulse and was pronounced dead.

I reminisce about Mel and his case often. Today, there seems to be a disconnect between our understanding of what medical technology can offer and a consideration of the repercussions. Most of the time there is no single correct choice but sometimes doing less is better than doing more.

At other times, you wish you could offer more. Particularly for a person who has not yet arrived at old age.

~~~

Linda was a 64 year old woman who had been under my care for a number of years. I had been treating her for hypertension and chronic back pain. Gradually, she had shared stories of her personal life with me—her unhappy marriage, her desire to retire soon and find some enjoyment in life. She felt trapped in a loveless marriage, and described her husband as an uneducated man who thought he knew everything. According to Linda, he was emotionally abusive and drank to intoxication each night. She remained married because she believed she would not be able to survive financially on her own. While she was thorny around the edges, I liked her and we respected each other a great deal.

She seemed to enjoy debating every recommendation I made. Without any background in science or medicine, she would take me on. Once, after stents had been placed in her coronary arteries to prevent heart attacks, I said, "Linda now is a good time for you to start taking a statin medication, Lipitor. I can see that your cardiologist had recommended this as well."

"Well," she countered, "I don't think that is necessary."

"Why is that?" I asked.

"I don't follow the correct diet. So, I can change my diet and that will lower my cholesterol. Problem solved."

"Linda, for 64 years you have been aware of low-fat diets. You have had many years to change your diet. How do you expect to do that now?" I asked.

"I just want more time to change. Besides, what are you basing your decision on?"

"Your total cholesterol is 249, your LDL cholesterol is 170, and your triglyceride level is over 200. The National Cholesterol Expert Panel guidelines, which are set by the foremost minds in the management of cholesterol, recommend those patients who have had a myocardial infarction or who have had cardiac stents placed need to have LDL cholesterol of less than 100 for starters. In all my years in practice, only 10 patients out of over 100 ever got close to this type of reduction without medication."

"Well, I think I can, besides there are side effects—I could damage my kidneys," she offered.

If I didn't like Linda so much I would have been getting annoyed with this debate.

"Statins can damage your liver, not your kidneys," I said. "In 25 years, I have had five patients experience minor *reversible* liver enzyme abnormalities. I repeat: *all reversible*."

"What proof do you have that these work anyway?" she asked.

With a sigh, I advised her that there had been over 10,000 patients enrolled in randomized double-blind placebo-controlled trials that had shown reductions in events of not only myocardial infarction but also strokes and deaths when LDL cholesterol are lowered to levels below 100.

"Well, I need more time. I don't trust these studies anyway. I'll think about it. I also don't ever listen to the cardiologist because he doesn't listen to me" she added.

Linda had been a heavy smoker for decades, grudgingly quitting only when she needed coronary artery stents to prevent her from having a major heart attack. As one aliment would simmer down, a new one would surface. Her heart scare was followed by lumbar spinal stenosis—a painful bulging of the lower (lumbar) disks in the spine.

Stenosis is the medical term for narrowing in and around a given structure. Spinal stenosis is a condition in which narrowing of the spinal cord results in pinched nerves in the spine. It is degenerative, causing the narrowing of the spinal cord, nerve root canals and joint spaces between the vertebrae of the spine caused by bone and ligament overgrowth in local, segmental or generalized regions. The result is a compression of spinal nerves and nerve roots. Lumbar spinal stenosis leads to persistent pain in the buttocks, a lack of feeling in the lower extremities and, not surprisingly, decreased physical activity. The most common cause of the degeneration is age, which is why spinal stenosis occurs in virtually the entire adult population; it is part of the natural aging process. Symptoms can include pain while standing or walking; lower extremity weakness resulting in poor coordination and balance; loss of sensation in lower extremities; and sometimes problems with bowel or bladder function.   Concurrently it is estimated that over 400,000 Americans, mostly over the age of 60, may be suffering from lumbar spinal stenosis. As a matter of fact, the most common reason for surgery in persons over 60 in the United States today is lumbar spinal stenosis. This number will grow as Baby Boomers age.

Treatment for spinal stenosis ranges from the most conservative, such as avoiding activities that could aggravate the condition, application of ice or moist heat, and loss of excess weight. Canes and walkers might also be suggested for individuals with balance problems. Physical therapy is often prescribed to build strength and endurance, maintain flexibility of the spine, improve balance and control of pain. Medications such as tricyclic antidepressants, antiseizure medication, and narcotics can be prescribed. Steroid injections (also known as epidural spinal injections, ESI) have become commonplace in medicine today. An ESI can be given by a number of specialists including neuro or orthopedic spine surgeons, radiologists, and anesthesiologists. (Obstetricians do *not* deal with this condition. My father had lumbar spinal stenosis. Once, at a social gathering, when I introduced him to a friend of mine who was an obstetrician, Dad asked—much to my embarrassment—if he could perform his ESI, going on to say he was aware that a similar type procedure was performed during childbirth. My friend politely told him this procedure was not part of his specialty.)

An injection of a corticosteroid/cortisone into the spine near the point of the constriction can help reduce the inflammation and relieve some pressure thus resulting in diminished pain. There are limitations in the number of injections within a year's span, however, to avoid other possible side effects. Surgery may be an alternative if more conservative options are not effective in reducing discomfort.

To help alleviate Linda's pain, I referred her to a pain management specialist for epidural injections. In addition, I prescribed narcotics to complement the effect and ease her pain. I believed that her spine disorder might have been amenable to surgery but she steadfastly refused to consider that as an option, remarking, "I could end up paralyzed. I would never even consider that as an option."

This would soon become a moot point.

Linda's visit to her cardiologist was "routine," scheduled. While her cardiologist was a fine clinician, Linda found him to be "a rude, arrogant, condescending man." (Frankly, his behavior toward me, a colleague, was no better, and he never gave me the courtesy of a consultation discussion no matter how serious her condition had become.) I learned of the visit when the lab work from the cardiologist's office was forwarded to me. The results: chemistry profile was normal, cholesterol was elevated (as usual), and her complete blood count (CBC) revealed that she had developed anemia.

Anemia is the condition in which the number of red blood cells in the blood is low. Blood is comprised of two parts: a liquid part, called plasma, and a cellular part. The cellular part contains several different cell types. One of the most important (and the most numerous) are red blood cells. The others are white blood cells and platelets.. The purpose of the red blood cell is to deliver oxygen from the lungs to other parts of the body.

Red blood cells live about 100 days, so the body is constantly trying to replace them through a series of complex and specific steps. They are made in the bone marrow, and when all the proper steps in their maturation are complete, they are released into the blood stream.

When I discuss anemia with my patients I describe the bone marrow as if it were an automobile manufacturing and assembly plant. It is dependent upon raw material (iron and Vitamin B12), a production team (the bone marrow), and production orders, which come from various places (particularly, the kidney).

Having the correct number of red blood cells requires cooperation among the kidneys, the bone marrow, and nutrients within the body. If the kidneys or bone marrow are not functioning properly, or the body is poorly nourished, normal red blood cell count and function may be difficult to maintain. If we use my automobile plant as an example, when union workers (bone marrow) go on strike, cars cannot be manufactured. When the Tsunami hit Japan in 2011, the auto parts (raw materials) became scarce and production of new cars was reduced. When our economy becomes weak, there are fewer orders for production (blood counts fall). This all has to do with production, but certain diseases can cause a loss of blood, which is another way in which anemia can develop. When someone loses blood from a bleeding ulcer or a stabbing, for example, it is as if someone is stealing cars from the manufacturing plant.

Anemia is actually a *sign* of a disease process rather than a disease itself. It is usually classified as either chronic or acute. Chronic anemia occurs over a long period of time. Acute anemia occurs quickly. Determining whether anemia has been present for a long time or whether it is something new assists in finding the cause. This also helps predict how severe the symptoms of anemia may become. In chronic anemia, symptoms typically begin slowly and progress gradually, whereas in acute anemia symptoms can be abrupt and more distressing.

We need to determine if a low red blood cell count is being caused by *increased blood loss* of red blood cells *or* from *decreased production* of them in the bone marrow.

In the United States, 2 -10 percent of the population has anemia. Young women are twice as likely to have anemia as young men because of regular menstrual bleeding. Anemia occurs in both young and old, but in older people it can be more difficult to diagnose because, typically, older people have additional medical problems and those symptoms can obscure the picture the doctor is trying to examine.

In general, there are three major types of anemia, classified according to the size of the red blood cells: If the red blood cells are smaller than normal, this is called microcytic anemia. The major causes of this type are iron deficiency (low level iron) anemia and thalassemia (inherited disorders of hemoglobin). If the red blood cells size are normal (but low in number), this is called normocytic anemia, such as anemia that accompanies chronic disease or anemia related to kidney disease. If red blood cells are larger than normal, then it is called macrocytic anemia. Major causes of this type are pernicious anemia and anemia related to alcoholism.

A number of conditions cause anemia. Common causes of anemia include active bleeding such as loss of blood through heavy menstrual bleeding, or wounds. Gastrointestinal ulcers or cancers such as cancer of the colon may slowly ooze blood and can also cause anemia.

Because a low red blood cell count decreases oxygen delivery to every tissue in the body, anemia can cause a variety of signs and symptoms. It can also worsen almost any other underlying medical condition. If anemia is mild, it may not cause *any* symptoms. If anemia is slowly ongoing (chronic), the body may adapt and compensate for the change; in this case there may not be any symptoms until the anemia becomes more severe.

Symptoms of anemia can include fatigue, decreased energy, weakness, shortness of breath, lightheadedness, palpitations (a feeling of the heart racing or beating irregularly), cold skin, and a loss of "color" in the complexion. When anemia is severe, it can cause chest pain, angina, or heart attack, dizziness, fainting, and rapid heart rate. A change in stool color (black or maroon colored stools that are foul smelling), or visibly bloody stools can also be signs of anemia.

The low red blood cell count reflected in Linda's CBC would certainly explain why she told the cardiologist she was tired and more short of breath than usual. But before I was able to discuss the abnormal lab tests with Linda, her cardiologist had performed a heart catheterization—a diagnostic procedure to determine the extent and nature of the heart disease. He detected a narrowing in her coronary arteries and recommended open heart coronary artery bypass* as the preferred treatment option. As is standard practice, the cardiologist had injected an extra dose of dye to evaluate Linda's aorta, and had detected another abnormality, an aortic aneurysm* of approximately 6cm. If not treated, an aneurysm of this size would likely rupture within the next three to four years. The cardiologist also ordered a chest X-ray and the result (which was abnormal) was sent to my office as well. Now, a *fourth* problem had been detected in this woman, all within a week: a 6 cm lung mass, most likely cancer. I called Linda to see how she was feeling and to learn what she had been told by the cardiologist who had ordered all the tests. She was delighted that I called and indicated that no one had given her any of the test results, although the cardiologist had told her she needed heart bypass surgery and that her aneurysm would need to be repaired as well.

The drop in her red blood cell count was not only without explanation but also at a level that needed to be corrected before she had further adverse consequences. I arranged for her to have a transfusion, followed by a consultation in my office to review her overall condition and the test results. At the time of her transfusion, I ordered an additional blood test that confirmed that her anemia was most likely due to blood loss. Anemia from blood loss (also know as iron deficiency anemia) is very common and the likely cause for a woman of this age is bleeding from the upper digestive tract from an ulcer, or from her lower digestive tract from diverticulosis or, worse, colon cancer.

Linda already had some understanding about anemia as, coincidentally; I had treated her husband with a similar problem just two months earlier. His anemia, iron deficiency, was the result of blood loss from a bleeding stomach ulcer. The likely culprits for him were cigarette smoking, consuming a dozen beers day, and taking aspirin on a daily basis for his neck pain.

An ulcer in the digestive system is an area where tissue has been destroyed by gastric juices and stomach acid. Peptic ulcer disease is a general term for ulcers that occur in the stomach or duodenum (upper part of the small intestine). A peptic ulcer is an erosion or sore in the wall of the gastrointestinal tract. The mucous membrane lining the digestive tract erodes and causes a gradual breakdown of tissue. This breakdown causes a gnawing or burning pain in the upper-middle part of the abdomen. Although most peptic ulcers are small, they can cause a considerable amount of discomfort. Peptic ulcers are a very common condition in the United States and, as a matter of fact, throughout the world.

In the United States, an estimated 25 million people will suffer an ulcer at some point. That's 1 in 10 people. About 4 million people are affected by ulcers at any given time. There are approximately 350,000 to 500,000 new cases every year and more than 1 million result in hospitalization. Hospitalization for an ulcer? That may surprise you, but complications can be serious, causing death in about 6,000 people a year. Ulcers can occur at any age, although they are rare in children and teenagers.

Duodenal ulcers usually first occur between the ages of 30 to 50 years and are twice as common in men as in women. Stomach (or gastric) ulcers usually occur in people older than 60 years and are more common in women. Some of these ulcers turn out to be cancers.

We have learned a lot about ulcers in the last 20 years and, thankfully, effective therapies are now available. Researchers realized that people with ulcers had an imbalance between acid and pepsin, and the digestive tract's ability to protect itself from these harsh substances. Studies performed in the 1980s showed that up to a third of ulcers are actually caused by infection with a bacterium named *Helicobacter pylori*, usually referred to as *H pylori*. The H. Pylori bacteria are found in the stomach, where the bacteria are able to penetrate and damage the lining of the stomach and duodenum. Many people who are exposed to the bacteria never develop ulcers. Infection with *H pylori* occurs in all ages, races, and socioeconomic classes. It is more common in older adults, although it is thought that many people are infected in childhood and carry the bacteria throughout their lifetimes. It is also more common in lower socioeconomic classes because these households tend to have more people living together, sharing bathrooms and kitchen facilities. It is important to distinguish between ulcers caused by *H pylori* and those caused by medications only, because the treatment is completely different.

Aspirin, nonsteroidal anti-inflammatory drugs (such as ibuprofen and naproxen), and newer anti-inflammatory medications (such as celecoxib [Celebrex]), alcohol, caffeine, cigarettes, and radiation therapy (used in cancer treatment) can all cause ulcers. In addition, stress—both physical and emotional—can contribute to ulcer formation.

Elderly people with arthritis are especially vulnerable for ulcers as a result of the anti-inflammatory medications they take. People who have had ulcers or intestinal bleeding before are also at higher-than-normal risk.

Linda was to come see me a few days after her blood transfusion. I had spent several hours contemplating her case and how I was going to tell her all the details along with some very bad news. I asked my staff to allot more time than usual for me to spend with her and to schedule the appointment at the end of the day so that I would have adequate time to answer the many questions I anticipated she would ask. As I focused on her list of problems, I encountered a mosaic of medical scenarios. Here was a 64 year old woman with a multitude of devastating conditions occurring simultaneously: lung cancer*, severe three-vessel heart disease, a large abdominal aortic aneurysm and an anemia from a stomach ulcer (from consuming too much ibuprofen) or from a cancer somewhere in her gastrointestinal tract.

Before I entered the exam room, I took a deep breath and reviewed what I would say to her. Linda and her husband were seated, waiting calmly for me. She was thumbing through a *Southern Living* magazine and he was reading an old paper-back book. What was unusual was her husband's presence; he had rarely accompanied her. It had always been her preference to come alone.

The dynamics were different with Roger there; the intimate relationship I had with Linda alone was now complicated by the presence of a man she professed to despise. I was off-balance. I had to regain my composure without letting either one detect how I felt. I needed my game face. *You can do this,* I told myself. But I needed to reorganize my thoughts. I needed to be prepared for the barrage of antagonistic questions I anticipated from her husband. *He could care less about her. Why is he here,* I wondered. It would be inappropriate for me to inquire.

We made small talk for a few moments and then, in typical fashion, Linda said, "Doctor, stop beating around the bush and just tell me what's wrong with me." Since we had spoken over the phone before her transfusion, she was not completely uninformed about the anemia.

"Linda, I have a lot of test results to review with you but I want first to ask you some questions. Your answers will help clarify some things. Please, tell me about the chest pain and shortness of breath you have been experiencing." She told me she'd been short of breath for several months but had failed to tell me about it because she was smoking again and knew I would be disappointed. She grinned and gave out a deep cough.

I took another deep breath, looked directly at Linda and spoke with an authoritative voice, "Linda, I have several different tests to review with you today." I shot a glance at her husband as if to tell him, *Do not interrupt, she is the patient here.* I turned my attention back to Linda. "I've given this conversation a great deal of thought and I have a certain order I want to follow to make it as understandable as possible." I was going to begin with the end in mind.

"Linda, the news is bad," I said, being certain to be unequivocal. "First, I want to tell you that you have become severely anemic. At the moment I don't know why. It might be related to the medications that you are taking, namely Plavix and Aleve."

These two medications interfere with the action of platelets. She took Aleve to help relieve her back pain, and the Plavix was to keep her heart stents open so clots would not form and cause her to have a heart attack. Since she had already been given a transfusion (and, following my suggestion, she was no longer taking Plavix or Aleve), I told her a stool sample would be helpful.

"As bad as the anemia is, it's not the most serious problem at this time." She nodded her head. She was aware of the AAA and her coronary artery occlusions.

Her husband was on the edge of his chair. He wanted to add his two-cents. "Doctor, I had anemia and you just gave me a transfusion and I got better. When will she see a gastroenterologist? Shouldn't she be scoped, just like you did to me?"

He had started off by trying to appear interested but he really just wanted to show-off and ended up by saying something about himself. I didn't detect any sincere concern in his questions. He seemed detached, void, and without emotion.

Roger's interruption was like a ringing cell phone in a movie theatre during the opening scene of a murder mystery. It was challenging to regain focus. I had come into the room with an idea of what I would say. Although I always try to prepare for questions, distractions, or other changes in the direction of the conversation, it is inevitably difficult in such settings to anticipate how a person will react. Some families are united when they receive bad news while others become splintered. What is Linda's reaction going to be? Can I count on Roger to provide any nurturing? Linda has one daughter with whom she is very close; she is not present but I will expect her to be supportive. At least Roger was in the room to *hear* everything. There would be less of a chance he would later second-guess me.

My next task was to address the finding made by her cardiologist. I told her that as bad as her coronary arteries were they could be managed with medication and that her symptoms might have been exaggerated by her anemia. As long as her low blood count was corrected, her coronaries would not be a problem—for a while.

"What do you mean, 'for a while'?" she asked.

"Linda, the aneurysm is not likely to rupture in the very near future; it's unlikely to be a problem at all for at least another six months."

Her jaw dropped slightly. "You mean there's more?"

I knew that once I told her about the abnormality seen on her chest X-ray, she and her husband would be completely focused on that; there would never be a chance to answer any of her other concerns. I stopped and offered to answer any of her questions on the information I had provided so far.

For the next few minutes, I addressed her concerns about how these three problems could be handled. I told her that as long as her blood count remained stable we could assume that the drop in her count could well be explained by the combination of Aleve and Plavix and as long as they were not resumed there should not be much of a problem. What I was really doing was positioning my discussion to focus on the abnormality seen on the chest X-ray. I believed that it was not only her most serious condition but the one that was ultimately going to be the cause of her death. I wanted all of her questions answered before giving her the really bad news, because once we started talking about a lung mass and cancer, her rational brain would stop working.

The time had come. I took yet another deep breath and said, "I have information about your chest X-ray that I want to discuss with you."

"You mean you have more bad news for me," she said, no longer trying to hide her trepidation.

"Yes, I'm sorry, Linda, I do. There is a mass in the left side of your chest, in your lung. It was seen on the X-ray," I told her.

"How big?" she asked.

"Six to seven centimeters," I answered without showing much emotion.

"Are you telling me that in addition to anemia, a heart problem and an aneurysm, I also have a lung mass?"

"Yes" I said.

"How bad is it?" she asked.

"Very bad, I am afraid" was my terse answer. I had never had a case like this before.

She asked, "Where do we go from here?"

Primary lung cancer forms in the lung tissue, usually in the cells lining air passages. The two main types of cancers, small cell lung cancer and non-small cell lung cancers, are diagnosed based upon the appearance of cells under a microscope. Most lung cancers are non-small cell type and these are further subcategorized. Sometimes, people will have cancer from another part of their body travel or metastasize to their lungs. This is called secondary lung cancer, because the lungs are secondary compared to the original, primary location of the cancer. Secondary lung cancer is not lung cancer but rather the type of cancer from its original site such as breast or colon cancer. Such cancers are treated differently than primary lung cancers because it's a different disease.

When a lung cancer is diagnosed, the pathologist assigns it a type (either non-small cell lung cancer or small cell lung cancer) and then assigns a stage to the cancer. The stage is a formal classification that signifies the extent of the cancer and determines the treatment offered to the patient. Lower stage numbers signify less advanced cancers; for example, a stage I is an early-stage cancer and most likely will have not spread from its original place of origin. The stage IV cancer indicates an advanced stage cancer and may appear in the lung as well as other areas of the body (metastases).

Lung cancer is one of the most common cancers. In 2007, lung cancer accounted for approximately 15 percent of all cancer diagnoses yet 28 percent of all cancer deaths. It is the second most diagnosed cancer in men and women (after prostate for men and breast cancer for women). *It is the number one cause of death from cancer each year in both men and women.* Because lung cancer can take years to develop, it is mostly found in older people—as a matter of fact, the average age of a person diagnosed with lung cancer is 71. Overall, lung cancer affects men more than women, but the gap is closing. It is well recognized that cigarette smoking is the cause of most lung cancers but there are other risk factors. Exposure to asbestos, radon, environmental toxins and secondhand smoke can cause lung cancer as well.

I paused for a moment to allow Linda to regain her composure. The implications of what I had just told her were devastating. I had enough experience with lung masses of this size and location to realize she had a very limited life expectancy and the mass would turn out to be an advanced stage of lung cancer. I could tell by its location that it most likely extended beyond the lung proper and was touching the chest wall. My suspicion was confirmed when she told me that it hurt her when she took a deep breath, a symptoms suggesting that the tumor was rubbing against the inner chest lining, the pleura. At this point she was beginning to realize, just as I had a few days earlier, that none of the other problems we had previously discussed mattered very much at all. I remained focused on the end, which from my standpoint meant confirming the diagnosis and setting a course of action.

"I will do anything you want, Linda, to confirm the diagnosis—that this is really a cancer—and to control whatever pain you may have. I want to send you to the hospital, where the radiology department can have the mass biopsied."

"Do I really have to, Doctor? You know what we are dealing with," she replied.

What would a visit with Linda be like without some type of objections? I thought to myself. "Linda," I exclaimed, "getting the biopsy result will confirm what we are dealing with and allow me to provide you with a more realistic prognosis, and I know you really want that. Neither you nor I want to be in a position a few months from now where we question the diagnosis," I added.

She agreed. Her husband sat pensively in his chair, wanting to interrupt. Each time he cleared his throat before attempting to speak, I shot him a glance: this was his wife's life we were talking about and he was not to interrupt her. She would make her own decisions.

Arrangements were made for a biopsy of the mass. We agreed we would get back together to discuss the next steps. It was understood that I would present her with various treatment options including no treatment at all. To be perfectly clear she really had no viable options. The lung cancer—if indeed that's what the mass was—was going to be the cause of her death, and I was certain she had less than 6 months to live. It was, however, important for her to have input into all the medical decisions. At this point, I felt I had given her enough information. Now she could mull it over for the week or so before our next visit when we would discuss the result of the biopsy. As we left my office, she said, "Thank you for being so honest with me, Doctor, and for taking so much time to explain this to Roger and me." I touched her on the shoulder as she walked down the hall, and gave her a reassuring glance. "You're welcome, Linda. I am sorry I had to give you such news but I certainly prefer to do it myself rather than have someone else speak to you about it." Her husband Roger looked at me, extended his hand and said, "Thank you, Doctor, for spending so much time explaining this to us today. We really do appreciate it."

When Linda, Roger, and I got back together 10 days later, the discussion revolved around the biopsy and what treatment options were viable for her.

"The results confirmed my suspicion. It is an adenocarcinoma, a type of non- small cell cancer. This is one of the most common forms of lung cancer and it is so large it is touching the chest wall, making it a Stage IV."

Her husband, Roger, silently nodded his head as if to acknowledge that this was the diagnosis he was expecting. He was stone-faced and somber.

Linda spoke up. "Well, I am not surprised based on the information you gave me at the last visit, Dr. Bernstein. What do we do next?"

I let out a big sigh. She had accepted what I had to say and was now looking for some guidance. This was a tremendous accomplishment considering the huge burden of information she had received just ten days earlier.

"Management of your cough and pain control are the most important issues right now. I also want to make sure you understand the consequences of your condition," I told her.

She acknowledged that she understood, but did seem to want to refresh her understanding about her heart condition and her aneurysm. (I sometimes refer to this as "reviewing the bidding"). In a very frank and understanding tone I reassured her that she had little to worry about with regard to those conditions. Still, she pressed the issue as had always been her style.

"But Doctor, I am still wondering about my aneurysm and my stents. What will we do about them?"

I opened my eyes wide and looked at her in silence as if to say, *Don't make me rehash the bad news I gave you last week, only to return to the fact that they do not matter at all.* She got the message.

Over the next few visits, I prescribed medication to suppress her cough, reduce her pain and address her poor appetite. I arranged for Linda to be enrolled in Sun Coast Hospice, knowing it would help her with pain management and the loneliness of her loveless marriage. She knew I understood what was going on in her marriage and was grateful. She died six weeks later, peacefully, at home, with her daughter at her side. Roger's presence always seemed awkward. In a way, at the time of her death, Linda was able to disengage emotionally from him, like a caged bird being set free. He could no longer burden her.

A few weeks after Linda died, I ran into her daughter at a professional networking gathering. She gave me a big hug and expressed her gratitude for the manner in which I had cared for her mother. "The Hospice team was wonderful. Mom died with dignity, in the comfort of her own home." Tears welled up in my eyes. I was touched and speechless.

~~~

The reader is entitled to wonder at this point if any of my cases have favorable outcomes. The answer is, *Yes, many do.* (Sometimes, as a geriatrician, I'm more surprised at this than the patient.) As a matter of fact, I have decades-long relationships with most of my patients My medical approach of beginning with the end in mind does not mean I spend my days sharing one piece of bad news after another. Rather, it is a way to keep a person's overall health and way of life at the front of my thoughts as varied diseases, illnesses, or injury take their toll and diagnostic reports pile up in thick manila folders (or, nowadays, in electronic files). Even when I treat hypertension, for example, or diabetes or high cholesterol—conditions that, on their own, can be very successfully treated today—I am always planning with the end in mind. The end goal, in those cases: prevention of a heart attack, stroke, or death.

~~~

When my patient, Roberta, fell and fractured her hip, she was an 82 year old widow who lived alone and enjoyed her independence. A retired school teacher, she took pride in keeping herself fit. She played tennis regularly (with much younger women), and was on the court when she fell. When one of her 50-year old tennis buddies came to the hospital to visit, she was astonished to learn how old Roberta really was.

The challenge I faced with Roberta was exactly what made her so unique in the first place: her independence. Once her hip was repaired she would need time in a rehab facility but what would she do after that? Her son lived in Chicago and had, as she would frequently remind me, "his own life with a job and family." He could not be expected to move to Florida, even temporarily, to care for her—nor did she want him to. This is a common refrain I hear from patients.

I discussed the options with Roberta, her social worker, and her son. She was lying in her hospital bed with her right leg tied to a weighted device (called Bucks traction) holding it in place.

"Roberta, tomorrow you will be taken to the OR to have your hip fixed. The surgeon tells me that he has to make just one small incision and place two special screws in your leg to hold the broken pieces in place," I explained.

"How long with that take?" she asked.

Patients always ask that question, as if they have an appointment later in the day they cannot afford to miss (like getting their nails done or catching their soap opera). "About an hour, or less," I told her.

"I am worried about the screw, Doctor. Can they come loose? You know I want to return to playing tennis and I cannot play with a loose screw," she exclaimed.

"Now, Roberta, let's take one step at a time. Let's set some goals."

"Good idea. When can I get home?" Roberta asked.

This was where things could get sticky.

"My plan is for you to return home with complete independence but first we have to set some intermediate steps. You will go home after your have fully recuperated at the rehab center and can get out of bed independently. You can't go home without a plan for assistance with some of your daily activities, like cooking, cleaning and shopping. You'll have to find someone to take you places too, for things such as grocery shopping and getting to your salon to get your hair done," I explained. These were two activities that I knew were an important part of Roberta's routine.

"How long will that take?" she asked.

"Three to six weeks," was my quick answer.

She was starting to understand the true impact her fall was having on her life as she liked to live it. "So, how long will I remain in the hospital and how will I get to the rehab facility?"

I explained that her hospital stay would be three days, after which arrangements would be made for her to be transported to the rehabilitation facility. I deliberately kept my tone confident, and told Roberta I had seen the kind of injury heal well many times before. Her son sat on a chair near her bed, acting like a spectator at a tennis match as Roberta and I exchanged volleys. Together, she and I eventually agreed on the goals and put together a plan that would allow her to return home and resume her independent life as quickly as possible.

"Once you're back in your apartment, you will still need some level of home health care for awhile. We want to make sure you continue to heal and the assistance is part of that plan," I emphasized. I knew from experience that as Roberta regained her strength, she would be at risk of an additional injury, including a fall.

Roberta was a great success story. She sailed through surgery, made rapid strides at the rehab center, and was back in her apartment in six weeks. She balked briefly about having the home health providers checking in on her but soon appreciated the help and companionship. Three months after surgery, she had returned to her independent way of life. She has not resumed tennis yet but she does bowl once a week. On her last visit to see me, she told me of her upcoming vacation in Europe with her son.

~~~

I met Simone Crawford when I was asked to care for her husband, Larry, at the rehab center where I served as medical director. Larry was a challenge: he had Alzheimer's disease and had been transferred to the rehab center after suffering a spinal compression fracture. He became confused easily, and had required restraints while in the hospital. Now, he was unable to walk.

"Larry is broken, Doctor, and I hope you can fix him," was Simone's straightforward request when we first met. "I will do anything you tell me to get him up and out of that bed. I want him home," she finished.

At first, I found Simone demanding, not to mention unreasonable. How could she be in complete denial about the degree of her husband's dementia and immobility? She was clearly intelligent. It was as if she were blind. But, as I was to learn, Larry was simply the love of her life, and her devotion to him was fierce. They had been married for 57 years.

"I will do anything for him. If the tables were turned, he would do the same for me."

Over the course of my first few visits, I learned that Simone (who at 84 was only a year younger than her husband), was also responsible for caring for her 86 year old sister. The sister, who also had Alzheimer's, lived with Simone.

"Mrs. Crawford" (I still had a formal relationship with her at that time), " I have evaluated your husband's condition and although I realize you were able to take care of him before his fall, he now has so many things wrong with him that I don't even know where to start. I do not feel it is realistic for you to plan on *ever* taking him home."

Simone was unmoved. "I will show you, Dr Bernstein. I will get him home."   And she did. She proved me wrong; three months after his arrival, Simone took Lou home and continued to care for him and her sister all by herself. I don't know how she did it. His poor sleeping habits and constant repetition of questions had been a challenge for the rehab facility staff—years younger than Simone, and only caring for Larry in eight-hour stretches.

We had butted heads over her husband's prognosis but I must have done something to please Simone because soon after getting Larry home she asked me to take her as a new patient. She wanted to change doctors because she was displeased with the attention she and her husband had received from their prior physicians. As impressed as I was with her courage and optimism, I was reluctant; I had experienced her stubbornness firsthand.

At her first visit, I asked the usual questions a doctor asks to get to know a new patient. I listened with amazement as she detailed the role she played in managing her husband's care at home. I was honored she had chosen me to assume her care. Her prior physicians had reputations for being very bright (but not particularly empathetic).

When I began the physical exam, I expected to find a very fit elderly woman. She was, in every respect but one. As I held my stethoscope to her chest, I heard a loud heart murmur. *Whoosh, Whoosh, Whoosh.* I have been listening to heart sounds since I was a second year medical student and it's fair to say I listen to them all day long. Most of the time, the sound of the heart is crisp, a distinct but soft medium-pitched *lub-dub*. I hear murmurs frequently; they usually make a soft blowing sound, like when a person blows out a single candle. Simone's was different. It was loud and nasty. Like someone in a hurry to blow out 10 candles in one short loud, low-pitched breath. *Whoosh, Whoosh, Whoosh.* It was the sound of a badly leaking mitral valve. Her previous doctors could not have missed it. How was it that she had never been told about it?

The heart's mitral valve is located on the left side, between the upper chamber (atrium) and lower chamber (ventricle). It enables blood to flow from the left atrium into the left ventricle but not in the reverse direction. Heart valves work like one-way gates, helping blood flow in one direction between heart chambers or in and out of the heart. The mitral valve (so called because it looks like a bishop's miter or headdress) has two "flaps" (cusps).

When the mitral valve is damaged—for example, by an infection—it may no longer close tightly. This lets blood leak backward, or regurgitate, into the upper chamber. As a result of this leakage, the heart has to work harder to pump the extra blood and meet the demands of the body. Small leaks are usually not a problem. But more severe cases weaken the heart over time and can lead to heart failure, a leading cause of death in older Americans.

There are two forms of mitral valve regurgitation*: chronic and acute. Mild to moderate chronic mitral valve regurgitation may not cause any Symptoms, but moderate to severe disease can result in mild Symptoms for decades and later develop into heart failure. Symptoms of heart failure include shortness of breath with activity, which later develops into shortness of breath at rest and at night. Extreme tiredness and weakness can also be expected.

Acute mitral valve regurgitation is an emergency. Symptoms, which can include severe shortness of breath, fast heart rate, lightheadedness, weakness, confusion, and chest pain, come on rapidly. Because there may be no symptoms when the acute event occurs, a specific type of heart murmur may be the first sign of this condition. Further tests to check the heart include clarifying the nature of the condition. An electro-cardiogram (EKG, ECG) looks for abnormal heart rhythms. A chest X-ray is used to check heart size. An echocardiogram, which is a cardiac ultrasound, is employed to help to determine how serious the valve problem is. Finally, a cardiac catheterization is performed to see how serious the problem is and to look for coronary artery disease.

At the end of our first visit, I informed Simone of my findings.

"Simone," (we were now on a first-name basis), "you seem remarkably fit for your age or even for someone 10 years younger. I've discovered one problem, though, and it might be serious. I heard a murmur."

"Well, Doctor, I have never had a murmur," she said in her matter-of-fact style. "What can we do about it?"

I explained that what I had heard through my stethoscope concerned me. "This murmur sound like it represents a very leaky valve and is something that has occurred silently. If we don't address it quickly, you can suffer severe problems. I want to develop a plan," I said in a reassuring voice.

I ordered tests to evaluate the condition of her heart and in particular, her mitral valve. I knew I would have to put together a coherent plan that would include dealing with not only her damaged heart valve but also her husband's and sister's care while she was incapacitated. I did not want her worrying over Larry or anything else and adding to the tremendous anxiety that surrounded her diagnosis. The plan would *have* to include getting her home in a better condition than when she left for the hospital. The eventual return home was the "end" I focused on as, together, we considered her options. Within three weeks, Simone had an echocardiogram and consulted with a cardiologist and a heart surgeon.   It turned out Simone's mitral valve must have had an abrupt injury, causing a significant leak. Luckily, at the time I discovered it, her heart had not gone through any of the changes that a chronic leak would cause; it was still healthy and could be repaired with surgery. The valve was replaced, and Simone returned home seven days after surgery—a remarkably speedy recovery. With the help of her daughter and home health care nurses her recuperation was nothing short of miraculous. All these years later, she is still a patient of mine and a person who continues to impress me.

~~~

Notes on living longer:

- Beginning with the end in mind helps you and your doctor develop intelligent strategies for solving complex health problems.
- Establishing clear personal and health goals will help when you encounter the challenging events that are part of aging.
- It is important to establish a long-term relationship with a physician; don't wait for a health crisis to initiate the search for a primary care doctor. When you and your doctor get to know each other over time, you will be better prepared for complex discussion about your health and healthcare options.
- When you, your family, and your doctor share realistic expectations, you will be better prepared to face difficult healthcare decisions.
- Having a comfortable and trusting relationship with your personal physician can make even the most serious medical decision tolerable.
- Feel comfortable about asking for additional opinions. A good doctor will respect this request.
- When challenged by considerable data, sit with your physician and sketch out a plan that makes sense— begin with the end in mind.
- Make sure you understand how you and your healthcare team will get to the "end," your goal.
- Be certain to thoroughly understand how each test or medication choice gets you closer to your goal(s). Keep a notebook with your questions, your doctor's answers, and other pertinent information.
- Ensure that healthcare documents such as a Living Will, Health Care Surrogate Designation and Power of Attorney are up to date and in safe place (such as a

safe deposit box), and that all appropriate individuals (your spouse or other family members, your primary care physician, and your attorney) are informed of your intent.

- Discuss the content of your Advance Directives with your primary physician and be sure it is part of your medical record.
- Keep your Will up to date.

Resources and Links :

- Advance Directives:
  - o www.cancer.org/Treatment/ FindingandPayingforTreatment/Understanding FinancialandLegalMatters/AdvanceDirectives/index
  - o www.cancer.gov/cancertopics/factsheet/support/ advance-directives
- Healthcare Agents: Choosing One and Being One
  - o www.caringinfo.org/i4a/pages/index. cfm?pageid=3286
- Making Medical Decisions for a Loved One at the End of Life
  - o www.acponline.org/patients_families/pdfs/health/ med_decisions.pdf
- Five Wishes—Aging with Dignity
  - o www.agingwithdignity.org/five-wishes.php

Chapter 9

But Doctor, I Am a Good Driver!

*The elderly don't drive that badly; they're just the
only ones with time to do the speed limit.*

– Jason Love

My alarm clock awakened me at 6:00 a.m. on a Monday, the start of a busy week. My routine starts with hospital rounds, which usually takes 45 minutes to complete. I will then rush to the office to see patients until 4:30 pm. I'll have time to finish paperwork before attending a meeting that runs from 6:00 p.m. to 8:00 p.m.

As the day begins, I turn on the morning news, mainly to catch the weather. The morning meteorologist is an acquaintance of mine and it's nice to see someone I know at this hour. The breaking news for this morning is about a missing woman. The story immediately draws my attention. 'Is it one of my patients?' I ask myself. The news story revealed that an 86-year old woman who resides in a local adult retirement facility and who reportedly has Alzheimer's disease, yesterday took her car to run some errands and failed to return. The news anchor indicates that the police spent hours searching for her and that this morning a more aggressive search will ensue.

As I step into the shower I instinctively knew exactly what had happened to this woman. Since the car had not been found, nor was there any police or hospital report of accident or injury, she was either lost, as in hundreds of miles away, or had driven off the road and died. A few days later, my prediction was confirmed as I read the following headline in the St. Petersburg Times: *Woman, car, found in water.*

The article reported that the woman had moved to the area to be closer to her family and had been living in an adult retirement facility. The family has described her as very self-sufficient but she had had short-term memory problems and so for the first month after moving to the new community, they had taken away her car keys "until she settled in." After 30 days, the car keys were given back to her. Family reports indicate that she did not drive far. "She just ran a few errands. We never questioned her driving skills. We never had to have a conversation about how to take the car away because it never came up."

I was 16 years old when I learned how to drive and I got my license at age 17. My first car, a white 1966 Buick Skylark convertible, originally belonged to my mother and then my brother. It was 6 years old and perfect. I loved that car and because I was first among my friends to drive, I put on a lot of miles. My parents regarded it a privilege; to me it was freedom and independence. No longer would I have to rely on Mom or Dad to pick my up from a movie or a friend's house or to drive me to the train station. I was free. As I reflect upon my first experience diving and how elated I felt to be behind a wheel, feeling that sense of control and independence, I can assure you that the thought never crossed my mind that one day I might have to face giving up my license and losing my independence.

What seniors face when their driving skills progressively deteriorate underlines the bigger problems: their failure to recognize the loss of motor skill, reflexes, and visual perception, as well as any authority that would be so malevolent as to terminate their driving privileges. This age group never had to deal with terminating their parents' driving privileges because most of their parents did not live to an advanced age nor did they suffer the chronic diseases that today's seniors face. In other words, their parents died before their driving skills deteriorated. As a result, today's elderly were never faced with this particular problem.

Over my career as a physician, I have had to face this situation countless times and it is always a painful experience. This situation triggers tears, anger, and outright disregard for the law or others who share the roadways. When my children were young and I knew from my practice that these horribly unsafe drivers where on the local roads at the same time as my children, I felt *very* uneasy.

I recall the first encounter I had with a patient regarding the older-driver issues. It was with a man named William who was a retired Salvation Army officer. Between he and his wife, they had referred as many as 100 of their friends to my office. He and his family were extremely nice. Their referrals made up a major portion of my practice. I have never forgotten their kindness or their role in the growth and success of my practice.

William developed Alzheimer's disease in his late 70s and his wife, who was a strong and vital force in their marriage, assumed most of the day-to-day chores and thinking. Even though William had always been a kind and gentle man, had a stubborn streak and he became more quarrelsome. I did my best to manage his dementia in a time when there were no medications available to slow down the progression of this dreaded condition. As I watched the disease progress, I saw the toll it was taking on his wife, Phyllis. She would rely more and more on their daughter, who lived out of town.

It became apparent to me that William was still driving despite very poor short-term memory and his wife's claim that he was a dangerous driver. I knew I had to do something, but what? I had little experience with this sort of thing but lives were literally at stake if he continued to drive. His wife seemed powerless to do anything about the situation. Suddenly, I saw an opening: William had been having problems with his eyes and was seeing an ophthalmologist, who had recently told him that his eyes had deteriorated and he should no longer drive. Wow, just the break this wimp of a geriatrician was looking for—someone else told him not to drive and there was a medical reason for it. I sat back and relished the fact that I was not the one to terminate his privileges. What a relief. About one month later though, William arrived in my office with a giant smile and told me that the ophthalmologist had given him permission to drive again.

By this time, this usually pleasant man had become totally irrational when we discussed his driving. He talked in circles; he rationalized how important it was that he drove; he acted like a 5 year old. Suddenly I had a brilliant idea. I said, "William, may I see your license, please?" He opened his wallet and with great pride, took out the license and presented it to me. I felt like the devil as I looked at it. I complimented him on just how handsome he looked in the picture and slipped it into the pocket of my white lab coat. I took one look at his startled and sad face and realized just how crushed he was. He would never get his license back, never drive again. It was as if he lost his manhood. He was angry, but he did not yell or curse. I sent the license into the DMV with a letter requesting it be revoked due to his diagnosis, and thought that that was the end of it.

While he never drove again, he never forgot that "Bernstein took away my license." As his disease progressed and he lost his memory (and dignity), one thing he never forgot was, "Bernstein took away my license." I realized then that this approach, although effective, was not the proper way to terminate someone's driving privileges. I would like to believe I saved some lives by insuring that William was no longer behind the wheel, but I do wish I'd been able to accomplish that without causing him so much hurt.

Some months later, I was faced with a similar situation. Joe was a retired government lawyer from the Washington, DC, area. He and his wife lived comfortably on a government pension. They enjoyed ballroom dancing and participated in competitions frequently. They spent a lot of money on the clothes required for these competitions.

Joe suffered from Addison's disease and it appeared he had some type of connective tissue condition as indicated by the fact that his ears were pinned close to his skull and very hard. After treating him for many years he developed Alzheimer's disease. As is typically the case, he kept his memory and cognitive decline a secret from his wife; eventually, however, it became apparent to her as well. What I have observed and been told by my patients, is that when friends begin to notice signs and symptoms of dementia and the diagnosis is made, "they drop you like a hot potato." Fear that this would happen, the couple kept their secret to themselves, not even discussing this with their daughter. When this situation became clear to me, we had a thorough discussion about the disease process as well as a new medication that had just become available. I would start Joe on a drug called Cognex.

On more than one occasion I strongly advised him and his wife that driving at this point would be dangerous and that he should relinquish his license. Each time I brought this to their attention, he refused the advice and his wife continued to be supportive of him. Since I had been so unsure how to handle this issue with William a few years earlier, his disease progressed and he became even more belligerent on the topic, so I did not pursue the issue vigorously.

Some weeks later I received a call from his wife saying that her husband had been in a serious auto accident and was taken to the county trauma center. He had suffered a broken pelvis, a punctured lung, and a severe head injury. No one else was injured in the accident. He died 5 days later. While I was relieved that no one else was hurt, his wife was distraught with grief about her loss and was forever guilt-ridden that she had not followed my recommendation to relinquish his license.

After this event, I did some investigating and discovered there were options I had not considered.

I began my exploration by contacting one of my patients who had a long career at the DMV. She informed me that the DMV had a form that *anyone* could fill out and anonymously report an unsafe driver. When the DMV receives this report, they notify the individual and require him or her to submit a form to their doctor; the onus is on the physician then to verify whether the individual should be driving.

The doctor's opinion and involvement *are* important in this process. I hadn't felt I had the technical skill to determine whether someone could drive, however, my knowledge and clinical reasoning led me to believe that a patient with diminished physical and/or cognitive abilities behind the wheel of a car cannot be safe—for him or any one else on the road. I have used this form many times and while I have remained anonymous, many unsafe drivers have had their license revoked.

One of my patients, who was especially displeased with the treatment she received by the DMV, pleaded with me to do something to help her. She was unaware that I was the one who had reported her. My staff and I had observed several dents in her car and very erratic driving in the parking lot of our office building. Isabel, 90- years old at the time, suffered from severe shortness of breath upon exertion. She was a very independent woman, widowed three times. She was formerly from Michigan, and now lived alone; all family lived out of town. As Isabel spoke about her daily routine, she stressed her need to drive. She indicated that she needed a car to go to the store and to see me. She was a very stubborn lady, and very intent on keeping her license. Much to my surprise, she begged, pleaded and even behaved seductively toward me (despite the 40- year difference in our age!) to gain my support. I maintained my position and did not give in. I recommended that she contact a driving evaluation program at a St. Petersburg hospital where a trained occupational therapist would be able to determine her ability to drive safely.

One day, a few weeks later, she came to me with a proposal. She would agree to a driving evaluation and if they said that she couldn't drive she would accept things the way they were. If not, the DMV should reinstate her privileges.

Isabel proceeded with the driver evaluation and shortly after the report arrived at my office. My staff strategically placed the report on the large pile of mail and other forms that I review daily. Since I have a tendency to multitask, I have to admit, I was on the phone when I picked up the report and took a look at it. I began to laugh. The person on the other end of the phone could not understand what he had said that was so funny.

The following are verbatim excerpts from the report on Isabel's driving evaluation:

Driver Evaluation Summary
Date: 08/08/2006
Referring Physician: David Bernstein MD
Diagnosis: Cardiac Disease

<u>Part Medical History</u>: The patient is a 93-year old female with a history of heart disease.

The DMV medical advisory board is requiring this evaluation. The patient has a Florida driver's license valid through 2009 with no restrictions. She denies having any tickets or accidents on her record. She lives alone in a retirement community with no family available to provide transportation.

<u>In-Clinic Assessment</u>: She has functional range of motion, strength, and coordination for her age. Cervical range of motion is within functional limits for her age. She walks independently without assertive devices or gait deviation. Brake reaction times are acceptable. The test was completed with her right foot on the gas and her left foot on the brake, which is her usual style of driving.

<u>Perception</u>: Her far vision without correction is 20/40-2 on the right and 20/40-2 on the left and 20/40-1 with both eyes. She appears to have a visual field deficit on the right, but did have difficulty following the instructions for this. Visual reaction times were impaired. Visual motor sequencing was significantly impaired.

<u>Cognition</u> The patient is alert and oriented. She is a very active and independent woman. She is somewhat nervous and talkative, requiring occasional redirection to task. She did have some confusion and frustration with difficult tasks. She has poor roadside

recognition doing 20 percent on road sign identification; 25 percent on traffic laws and rules. Memory is impaired with 2 out of 5 correct responses in long-term memory and 1 out of 3 word recall after 5 minutes for short-term memory.

<u>On The Road Assessment</u>: The patient participated in a one hour supervised driving on a sunny day with dry pavements. She was able to transfer independently. She did sit on a pillow to improve her line of sight over the steering wheel. She did require verbal reminders to fasten her seatbelt and adjust her mirrors with some verbal cues for shifting gears. She used her right foot on the accelerator and her left foot on the brake. She occasionally put her right foot on the brake and depressed the brake when she intended to press the accelerator. Upon exiting the parking lot, she required verbal cues to perform visual check to the left before pulling out.

In residential, on light city traffic at speeds no greater than 30 miles per hour; the patient drove with frequent verbal and physical assistance required. She had a tendency to slow inappropriately almost to a stop at intersections and pedestrian crosswalks. However, she made frequent rolling stops and ran a stop sign on one occasion, failing to stop before turning right. She did look both ways at the intersections. She did make right and left hand turns correctly in residential areas, but was inconsistent in her turn signal use.

On 2 lane roads with traffic lights, she had frequent steering difficulties, drifting out of her lane multiple times. She was not aware of other vehicles having to move over to avoid her. On one occasion, she was driving in empty parking spaces, rather than in the traffic lane. She used her inside rear-view mirror only for lane changes and slowed significantly. She required verbal cues to move into the turn lanes appropriately. She stopped at a red light and looked both ways and then initiated a left turn while the light was still red and the evaluator had to use the training brake to prevent her from going through the red light. On another occasion, she required verbal cues to stop at a yellow warning light turning red. When she did make a left hand turn, she failed to stay on the right side of the median and the evaluator had to use her hand on the wheel and the training brake to correct this. She drove in a shopping center parking lot in the back entrance and drove in the wrong direction between angled parking spaces, but was able to pull into an angled parking space correctly.

The evaluation was discontinued at this time and the evaluator drove the vehicle back to the facility.

RECOMMENDATIONS: It is the evaluator's opinion that this patient is not a safe driver. She was instructed to stop driving from this point on. She was very disappointed with these results and repeatedly requested re-testing, or allowing her to continue to drive for 3 more months until she could settle her affairs. She verbalized intention to move back to Illinois, where she would be able to get her driver's license. She is provided with a list of alternative transportation resources. She did have a ride home with some neighbors. She had difficulty accepting the results of this evaluation and was very upset.

Thank you for this referral.

When Isabel returned to my office after the test she was a bit sheepish, playing down the report, telling me, "It was just a bad day and that the tester flustered me," but she really felt she did not do badly and she did not believe that she was as bad a driver as the report had indicated.

According to the Florida Department of Highway Safety and Motor Vehicles, research indicates that most people will outlive their driving ability by 10 years. The most at-risk driver is the one with cognitive impairment. The AMA regards the safety of older drivers as a public health issue and estimates that the per-mile fatality rate for drivers over 85-years old is nine times as great as drivers 25- to 69-years old.

Why is relinquishing a driver's license such a problem? Why are our elderly taking such risks, not only for themselves but their loved-ones and others on the road? What do they see when they look in the mirror? I have been pondering these questions for many years and continue to be amazed at the resistance I receive when the "Driving Subject" is broached.

In my years as a geriatrician, observing and studying the reactions and subsequent behaviors after a discussion on the topic of driving are not so surprising. Consider this: These seniors are fighting to maintain their independence. Their last bastion is their ability to drive. When they can no longer get back and forth to the doctor, grocery store, and hairdresser, they view life as being over. They might have to move to a retirement center in order to have transportation or even worse move to a different town or state to live near one of their children. This option is one most find totally unacceptable. Many of them might willingly take advice from one of their children about something or other, but not about giving up their driving.

Another major factor is the lack of precedence. The group of elders who are currently facing this issue all lived through the depression and WWII. People had cars during and after the depression but not nearly the number that had them after WWII. In the mid 1940's through the 1950's this group acquired their first car. As a group, they did not have to face their parent about relinquishing their driving privileges. For the most part, their parents did not have the life expectancy we have today so that particular confrontation did not take place.

When I ask my older patients about how they dealt with *their* parents regarding this issue, they frequently tell me that their mother did not drive so they faced only one half of the issue. Most of the time their father was still driving when he got sick or suffered a stroke and then just stopped. Therefore, this is the first generation of individuals who are facing this issue. Driving as a senior and the decisions that surround their continued safety, for themselves and others, is uncharted territory.

In a survey conducted among baby boomers, for Caring.com in partnership with The National Safety Council, investigators found that suggesting to parents that they stop driving was considered to be the most difficult subject for children to bring up with their parents— more difficult than discussing funeral wishes or selling their house! Thirty nine percent (39%) of those surveyed said they would not be comfortable discussing driving status with their parents. Of those surveyed, 25% felt that their parents should voluntarily impose some restrictions or safeguards on themselves.

The public transportation system in most cities in this country does not meet travelers' needs. Seniors are no different! They are "spoiled" in this respect; when they want to go somewhere, they just get in the car and go. The prospect of calling a cab, waiting to be picked up, is just unacceptable to them. Many do rely on friends for rides but express they do not like to impose and, as a result, they often become isolated or very dependent on others.

Solving this problem is difficult and requires a solid understanding of the personalities and needs of the individuals. Love and respect from children and friends is imperative, as is providing alternatives when the license is revoked and the car keys are taken. We have dangerous drivers on our roadways that are in total denial that they have lost the skill to drive safely, and they are unable to determine when to stop. As a society, we have been too timid to address this critical problem and as a result, lives are put in jeopardy every day.

The lessons here are serious. Over the next 20 years there will be an astounding growth in senior drivers in the United States. The population of adults over 75 years old will grow from 18 million to 31 million. Since the accident rate for drivers over the age of 65 is higher than any other group other than teenagers, this could account for 100,000 accidents in the next 20 years.

New approaches are being developed as information is gathered about the growing risk this population faces. The American Medical Association, in conjunction with the National Highway Traffic Safety Administration, has created a guide booklet for physicians who treat older drivers. *The Physician's Guide to Assessing and Counseling Older Driver* is available online at: www.ama assn.org/ama/pub/caegory/10791.html

As an aid to empower caregivers and families, The Hartford Financial Services group and the Massachusetts Institute of Technology has developed a 30-page booklet, *At the Crossroads*, which can be used independently or in a classroom to facilitate conversation about driving cessation.

If you have a loved-one whose driving skills are putting him or her and others on the road at risk, don't put off the conversation you know you must have. I hope you will also include the family physician in these conversations. We want to help.

Notes on living longer

- As adults age, driving skills deteriorate and seniors fail to recognize their loss of skill.
- A desire to maintain independence and the lack of public transportation in most regions of this country perpetuates driving despite loss of skills.
- Society has not developed methods to restrict driving of senior adults.
- As an aging adult, be cognizant of the loss of skill and find alternative means of transportation.
- As the child of an aging parent gently discuss this issue and help develop a plan for alternative living arrangements which provide transportation and allow prolongation of independence. Consider bringing the matter to the attention the patients health care provider.

Resources and Links:

Alzheimer's Association, _Driving and Dementia_, Alz.org, Driving and Dementia Resource Center Retrieved November 16, 2011 from http://www.alz.org/care/alzheimers-dementia-and-driving.asp

Alzheimer's Association National Board of Directors, approved September 2011, *Driving and Dementia* Retrieved December15, 2011 from *http://www.alz.org/documents_custom/statements/driving_and_dementia.pdf*

The Hartford Group, *Dementia and Driving: Understanding Dementia and Driving*
http://www.thehartford.com/advance50/dementia-driving

Chapter 10

Dad—Hospice

And in the end, it's not the years in your life that
count. It's the life in your years.
– **Abraham Lincoln**

One of the enticing aspects of practicing medicine has been how I have evolved as a person and as a physician. In medical school I learned the basics; during my internship and residency I consolidated my knowledge and have built on that base every day since. Early in any physician's career, it is difficult to face end-of-life decisions (all our patients are strangers to us at that point) but over time we get to know our patients well, and become more comfortable with the concept that life will eventually end.

That said, I don't think we are really ever prepared to have our parents die. I was in medical school when I first heard the word "hospice." The concept and acceptance of it was in its infancy in the medical culture then, but over the past 30 years it has become welcome in our society. During that time, I have learned where it fits into my practice of medicine and my personal philosophy as well.

Actually, hospice is a concept that has been evolving since the 11th century. It is a type of care and a philosophy of care that focuses on the palliation (the alleviation of pain) of a terminally ill patient's symptoms. Those symptoms can be physical, emotional, spiritual or social in nature. Hospice care focuses on bringing comfort, self-respect, and tranquility to the dying patient, with an emphasis on care not cure. With this knowledge and my own experiences as a physician, I explained to my mother, brother and sister how hospice could help my father when he became terminally ill.

My father's health had deteriorated quickly over a six week period. I was summoned by my sister to pay a last visit. I immediately made arrangements for the drive across the Florida Peninsula to get to him. As Dad's life was coming to and end, I watched as his labored breathing slowed. Earlier in the day he had been "wheezy" and "wet" and his respiratory rate was 20-22, (normal is 16). Now the rate slowed to 12-14, and then slowed some more. It was just the way I believe it should be: my father surrounded by his family—Mom, my brother Lewis, my sister Nancy and me.

We discussed going to dinner (we are always talking about our next meal), so why would this occasion be an exception. Should we go out or bring something in and eat at the bedside? We were indecisive, but it was getting past Mom's usual dinner time; we needed to decide. I noticed Dad's respiratory rate slowing even more. No surprise, the hospice nurse had recently given him 10mg of morphine sulfate under his tongue for comfort and to ease his labored breathing. At that moment I had a flashback to something my dad had said to me a long time ago about his experience with morphine. It had been given to him by the medics in the field after he stepped on a land mine in France during World War II. It was morphine that eased his pain during all those months he spent in the VA hospital as he recovered from the injuries he had sustained and eventually, from the amputation of his right leg.

Dad was an inspiring man. I credit him for instilling in me a sense of determination, telling me, "If you put your mind to it, you can achieve anything you want." I credit him for encouraging me to go to college and later, medical school. He was not a flashy man, he did not have to be; his accomplishments in life spoke volumes. Other events in his life instilled a sense of generosity and charity and he instilled those traits in his three children

Dad was born in 1917 in a peasant village outside Warsaw. When he was 5 years old, his father left the village for the US, leaving him behind with his mother and three other siblings to wait their turn to come to the US. It would be five years until they received a visa and the money to travel to America. With his family, he boarded a cruise ship and traveled in steerage to Ellis Island, where he entered the US. He and his family lived in impoverished conditions in a one-bedroom, five story walk-up on the lower East Side of Manhattan. Six years later Dad's hard working father died of a stroke leaving him at age16 as the male head of the household. Dad grew up fast and learned to perform odd jobs to help support his family. His oldest sister married and the next older one became a maid out of town. When WWII started, he was anxious to serve but as head of the household and with poor vision and flat feet, he had to wait his turn.

He worked his way up the ranks to sergeant and after training in England was sent to France to fight in the Battle of the Bulge. I remember him telling me that he thought walking behind a tank, stepping in its tracks, would be a safe way to avoid land mines. He was incorrect. He stepped on a mine in France in March of 1944 and was sent back to Paris and eventually to the US to recover. He spent the next 18 months recovering from several operations in VA hospitals. This was a defining time for my father, and it was during his recovery that he developed a determination to succeed at whatever he set his mind to do. It was also at the VA hospital that he became "half a doctor" as he would frequently say to me, applying bulky bandages and an ace wrap to the smallest of cuts and bruises I suffered as a boy.

After his discharge from the VA and the Army, he worked with other Veterans and the United Auto Workers union to lobby Congress to provide automobiles with adaptive devices for disabled veterans.

Determined to overcome another obstacle, he decided to learn how to ice skate. I believe he chose this activity precisely because it presented a profound challenge for a man with WWII-vintage right leg prosthesis; if he could learn this he could do anything else he tried in life. It did prepare him for life with a prosthesis. This was the attitude that enabled him to deal with any obstacle he faced in life.

From his example, my siblings and I learned that if our father could "do it" (learn to ice skate with his wooden leg) there were no obstacles too large in *our* lives, only opportunities to face our own fears. We could achieve whatever goals we set for ourselves.

Dad struggled with his health most of his adult life. While he did have complications from his WWII injuries, most of his medical problems were related to hypertension, diabetes and high cholesterol. He was treated with medications in the 1960s and 1970s that we now consider archaic. They were difficult for him to tolerate. Despite medical problems and the lack of an exercise program or careful diet, he lived into his late 80s. (I did observe over the years he had primary care physicians who were competent and whom he trusted; he did not always follow their instructions but he respected them and they knew and understood him.)

When he moved to a retirement community, he had to leave behind his physician of 18 years. His health deteriorated and he needed a strong force to direct his care but unfortunately he never found one. He visited several different primary care doctors but was never content. Dad thought he was still the boss and when his new physicians did not follow his instructions he would leave and try out someone else. Dad fragmented his care as well, seeing many different specialists. Sometimes he would go to a VA doctor and at other times one in his community. When he developed urinary problems and the urologist did not do what Dad wanted, he found another one in a different community.

The biggest problem was that none of his new physicians seemed to communicate with one another. When he suddenly developed an acute inability to pass his urine in the middle of the night, Mom took him to the hospital emergency room. A catheter was placed in his bladder and at six in the morning my 89-year-old father was sent home. One of his new urologists suggested (despite the fact that Dad was nearly blind and unable to balance himself due to his amputated leg) that Dad place a small tube in his bladder 3-4 times a day to help it drain. Within a few weeks, his bladder backed up and he developed kidney failure. While waiting in the emergency room, he suffered chest pains but it was not until the morning that one of his physicians determined he was also suffering from a heart attack (myocardial infarction). Dad needed surgery to help overcome the blockage in the flow of urine from his damaged kidneys to his poorly functioning bladder. After that surgery, he was never the same. No one was able to explain exactly what happened, but I suspect he had suffered a stroke during the procedure. He never returned to his normal mental capacity.

In the final six weeks of his life, he was seen by no less than 42 different physicians in two different hospitals and one rehab facility. He was unable to develop rapport with any of these physicians and every day his condition worsened. Dad had made it abundantly clear to me and the rest of the family that he did not want to be kept alive by any artificial means; when he was no longer able to function and enjoy life, he did not want to be a burden to his family or the health system. Placing him in a rehab facility was a decision made with a great deal of thought and debate within the family. We agreed to give Dad one last opportunity to recover from the illnesses he had been treated for in the hospital, a chance to return home to an independent life. But he developed congestive heart failure, and when it became clear that he would never return home or have any independence we respected his wishes and Advance Directives and enrolled him in hospice. Suddenly, he became acutely ill, probably suffering another heart attack and ended up in a hospital his primary care physician did not attend. An "on call" doctor, whom he did not know—a total stranger— admitted him to a third health facility and reviewed the case with our family. It became clear that my father had a very limited chance for survival. In keeping with his wishes, my family made a decision to change directions and asked that he be provided palliative care by the local hospice.

The National Hospice and Palliative Care Organization (NHPCO) defines palliative care as treatment that enhances comfort and improves the quality of an individual's life during the last phase of life. No specific therapy is excluded from consideration. The test of palliative care lies in the agreement between the individual, physician(s), primary caregiver, and the hospice team that the expected outcome is relief from distressing symptoms, the easing of pain, and/or the enhancing the quality of life. The decision to intervene with active palliative care is based on an ability to meet stated goals rather than affect the underlying disease. An individual's needs continue to be assessed and all treatment options are explored and evaluated in the context of the individual's values and symptoms. In hospice care, the individual's choices and decisions regarding care are paramount and must be followed at all times.

Hospice provides quality, compassionate care for people facing a life-limiting illness or injury. This kind of palliative care involves a team-oriented approach that provides medical care, pain management, and emotional and spiritual support expressly tailored to the person's needs and wishes. Support is also provided to the person's loved ones as well.

The focus of hospice relies on the belief that each of us has the right to die pain-free and with dignity, and that our loved ones will receive the necessary professional support to allow us to do so.

- Hospice care focuses on caring, not curing and, in most cases; care is provided in the person's home.
- Is provided in freestanding hospice centers, hospitals, and nursing homes and other long-term care facilities.
- Is available to patients of any age, religion, race, or illness.
- Is covered under Medicare, Medicaid, most private insurance plans, HMOs, and other managed care organizations.

Back at Dad's beside, I knew he was dying. Morphine was being given to comfort him again, this time as he struggled unconsciously for his last breath. His time on earth was running out. We did not say anything to one another; we all knew what was just a minute away. I was at the foot of the bed, holding onto the stump of Dad's amputated right leg. Nancy was to my right, holding onto Dad's left leg, Lewis was holding Dad's right hand and Mom was holding his right. What happened next was a most astonishing event. Mom leaned over and said to Dad, "Walter, do you remember the cruises we used to go on? Walter, do you want to go on a cruise?" There was a pause and then Mom said, "Walter do you remember the yellow sweater I was wearing when we met at the skating rink?" In all my years of hearing that Mom and Dad met at Rockefeller Center at the ice skating rink I had never heard about a yellow sweater. Mom must have looked great in that sweater and it might have been their special secret that they shared up to the end. Then Mom said, "Walter, do you remember that song we used to sing?" Mom began to sing, a song I had never heard her sing before. It was a special song they had shared, "The Liar's Song." As Mom finished, Dad took a deep rattling breath, and exhaled. It was his last. Lewis noted that Dad's final facial expression was one that he had seen many times before, when Dad had said all he intended to say: he pursed his lips and it was over.

We stood around the bed, tearful, before we slowly left him. I reflected on how peaceful his passing was and how fortunate I was to have been there. He had achieved what many patients tell me they want: to die with their family at their side, without tubes and IVs and doctor and nurses aggressively trying to prevent the inevitable.

Dad was a courageous man and he faced death with the same stoicism he faced life. I would never describe him as a "health nut" but he did stop smoking cigarettes when the surgeon General came out with the initial warning in the 1960s that cigarettes are harmful to your health, and he was attentive about regular visits to his physicians. He was adherent to nearly every medication prescribed to him. Until late in his life, he kept excellent rapport with all his doctors and followed their advice.

When he moved to a new community, things broke down; he was not able to find a physician he could trust or partner with and his health suffered for it. How ironic that he, the father of a geriatrician, could not find a doctor he trusted when he most needed one. What he did have was a family he loved and trusted who surrounded him as he took his final breath.

<u>Notes for living longer</u>

- Experiences in life have a profound effect and impact on how you live your life and can shape who you become and what you can achieve.
- A long-standing relationship and partnership with your physician is extremely important for continuity of care and understanding.
- Doctor-patient relationships built on mutual respect and trust can lead to a longer and healthier life.
- Build and maintain a strong relationship with your physician.
- Discuss/negotiate how you want your long-term care managed.
- Trust you physician or find one you can trust, accept the wisdom and follow directions.
- Understand the value of love, family and generosity in life.
- Develop a positive attitude about life and your fellow man.

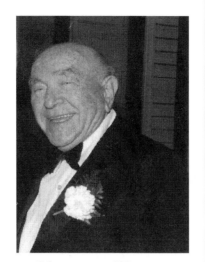

MY FATHER, WALTER

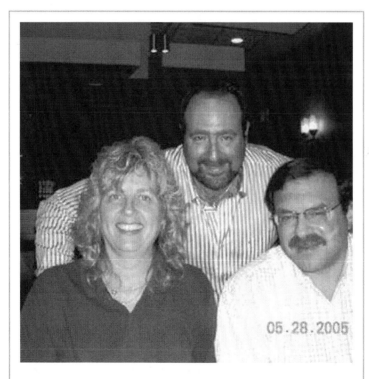

05.28.2005

MY BROTHER LEWIS, MY SISTER NANCY AND I HAD TO
MAKE DIFFICULT END OF LIFE DECISIONS

Resources and Links:

NIA.NIH.gov. (2011) *Talking to Your Doctor: A Guide for Older People*. Retrieved January 2, 2012 from http://www.nia.nih.gov/health/publication/talking-your-doctor-guide-older-people/getting-started-choosing-doctor-you-can

ElderparentHelp.com, *Selecting a Doctor*. Retrieved January 2, 2012 from www.elderparenthelp.com/healthcare/selecting-a-doctor

Hospice Foundation of America, http://www.hospicefoundation.org/

Suncoast Hospice, www.thehospice.org/

Chapter 11

Aunt Jeanette

When I was younger I could remember anything, whether it
happened or not.
– Mark Twain

As I boarded Southwest flight 347, bound for Ft. Lauderdale, I began reviewing my agenda for the weekend. I planned to attend a medical conference, spending the evenings on either side of it with my mother and sister. We were going to talk about my Aunt Jeanette's health. As the physician in the family I had been asked and agreed to tell this kind-hearted woman that she had a terminal and advanced cancer. The disease had been discovered during some recent tests ordered by her primary care physician. Complicating the situation was the fact that Aunt Jeannette had moderately advanced Alzheimer's disease.

All her life, Aunt Jeanette had maintained strong connections with her family. She had never lost her sense of humor, either, despite the challenges old age presented. She still laughed out loud at jokes and situations she found funny, which is unusual for someone with

Alzheimer's disease. During these past few years, she had found great pleasure interacting with a pet bird at her retirement home. That said, the staff there had reported that she had become more irritable lately, particularly when anyone tried to give her instructions. She still wanted to do things for herself, and was quite insistent about it.

As I looked out the jet window as we glided over the Everglades, I began to reminisce about this unique and wonderful woman. She was born in 1917 (the same year as my father) as one of four children raised by my maternal grandmother and grandfather. She married about the time I was born, and moved to Florida. I was told that the marriage "didn't take" and when I first became acquainted with her, she was living with my grandparents. I was one of her six nieces and nephews. We spent many Passover Seders and Thanksgiving dinners together until I went off to college and moved out of town. Later, she would travel to one home or another to participate in family gatherings. She was intelligent, a delight to have around and always made things fun. She had special relationships with each of us. Even Caesar, our pet Whippet, greeted her with enthusiasm as she entered our home because he knew he was in for a great walk with Aunt Jeanette. For Nancy, my sister, there would be endless games of Spit or Spite and Malice. My brother Lewis, the oldest of my siblings and the only one who remained in New York while Jeanette lived there, looked after her health and finances as she grew older and less able. When Aunt Jeanette moved to Florida, Nancy assumed that responsibility.

Everyone who interacted with Aunt Jeannette had a special story. I remember an occasion when Aunt Jeannette (who had never driven a car!) came along as I drove our family to Virginia for a wedding. I had a good set of directions and we arrived without incident. Coming home was a different story. I did not have a reverse set of directions and there were many intersections where I could turn right or left. I asked for help from the three people in the car. Dad, in the front seat, was not paying attention and his vision was very poor anyway. Mom was talking to my sister—*what a great time she had had!* And then there was Aunt Jeannette. She was in the back seat, giving me directions.

Needless to say, we wound up off course by 10 miles, ending up at Reagan Airport. At least I knew how to get back to the hotel from there.

Months later, Aunt Jeanette had the time of her life at my niece's Bat Mitzvah. She was in rare form. Well into her 80s, she danced and paraded around as if it were *her* party and the happiest day of life.

But soon after that fun occasion, Aunt Jeanette started to have health setbacks: heart ailments, arthritis and memory impairment, leading to her diminished independence. Eventually, she relocated to an ALF (assisted living facility) in Florida. Her family stayed close with a regular flow of visitors and she found a new friend (a bird!), that she spent time with each day. With the passing years her short term memory slipped more and more. She had always been very articulate and now was aware that she could not find words to express herself the way she wanted. She often repeated herself. She knew this and was frustrated by it. There was an element of fear about it also, as she was well aware of what Alzheimer's disease had done to her brother. As his disease progressed, he had become increasingly agitated and belligerent.

Another memory that came to mind as I sat back in my window seat was a party that was to be held for my mother. In the week before, Mom called Aunt Jeanette every day to remind her about the upcoming party. Jeanette was told what day and time it would take place. Mom would repeatedly remind her that lunch would be served, so she should skip the meal at her ALF and be prepared to be picked up in front of the building at noon. I arrived at noon to pick her up. But Aunt Jeanette was not in her usual position near the front door. I parked and went inside to find her. She was finishing her lunch! She sipped her coffee as I approached her. "Hi, *DAVID!*" (I always loved how she greeted me). She exclaimed, gave me a big hug, asking, "What are you doing here?"

I replied "I came to take you to Mom's party and *lunch.*" She looked at the two other people at the table, laughed and said, "I completely forgot and I have already eaten. I will be out in a minute. I just have to finish my coffee and this cookie."

Within the year, the staff asked us to disconnect the stove in her apartment because she would forget to turn it off, frequently burning something that left a foul odor permeating the hallways, not to mention exposing her and others to a risk of a fire. Aunt Jeanette was very disturbed about this additional loss of independence. The fact is, she really did not need to cook anything anyway, but she did like to make herself a cup of coffee or tea. My sister Nancy went out and bought her a microwave oven as a safer substitute.

Her next problem was hygiene. Aunt Jeanette had always been meticulous about her appearance. I was told that she started to have a foul odor about her, "like urine." The staff noted that there had been some incontinence. She had developed the habit of hanging her undergarments to air-dry them in her room. She told the staff that she had washed them but they discovered that she was skipping the washing phase, going directly to the drying phase. Oops!!

Before I continue my story about Aunt Jeanette, here are some salient facts and figures about Alzheimer's disease quoted from the Journal of Alzheimer's Association March 2012.

"Alzheimer's disease was first identified more than a century ago but research into its symptoms, causes, risk factors and treatment has gained momentum only in the last 30 years. Although research has revealed a great deal about Alzheimer's, the precise physiologic changes that trigger the development of the disease remain largely unknown. The only exceptions are certainly rare, inherited forms of Alzheimer's disease that are caused by known genetic mutations.

- Today, 5.4 million Americans are living with Alzheimer's disease −5.2 million aged 65 and over, and 200,000 under the age of 65. It is expected that by 2050, up to 16 million will have the disease.
- Of Americans aged 65 and over, 1 in 8 has Alzheimer's. Nearly half of people aged 85 and older have the disease.
- Another American develops Alzheimer's disease every 68 seconds. In 2050, an American will develop the disease every 33 seconds.

The warning signs of Alzheimer' are as follows:

- Memory loss that disrupts daily life.
- Challenges in planning or solving problems.
- Difficulty completing familiar tasks at home, at work or at leisure.
- Confusion with time or place.
- Trouble understanding visual images and spatial relationships.
- New problems with words in speaking or writing.
- Misplacing things and losing the ability to retrace steps.
- Decreased or poor judgment.
- Withdrawal from work or social activities.
- Changes in mood and personality."

The Symptoms of Alzheimer's disease creeps up upon a person slowly, insidiously devouring the persons mind without fanfare. Although the disease affects people in different ways, the most common symptom pattern begins with a gradually worsening ability to remember new information. This occurs because disruption of brain cell function usually begins in brain regions involved in forming new memories. As the damage spreads, individuals experience other difficulties. These are some symptoms that can be brought to the attention of a family doctor as an entry point for someone with memory impairment.

Alzheimer's disease afflicts older adults, naturally, as a geriatric physician I see it frequently. It is a sad part of my job to watch as people I care about deteriorate slowly before my eyes, particularly individuals I have known for many years. I also observe the effect it has on families, especially a spouse who becomes the caregiver by default. Whatever the stage of this horrible disease, they all had narratives of their own. Their families and friends went through what we experienced with Aunt Jeanette, doing the best they could.

Another sad truth is that as the individual loses his memory and cognitive ability he loses his friends and connections. As one of my patients told me, "No one wants to hang around or socialize with you when you cannot remember things." A spouse once said, "It is embarrassing to my husband and to me to see the expression on friend's faces when he repeats things over and over again."

I was brought back to reality as the intercom sounded…"*This is the captain speaking. We are approaching Ft. Lauderdale International Airport.*" The landing gear dropped, letting me know my weekend was about to begin.

A few weeks before my visit, Aunt Jeanette had awakened with redness in one of her eyes. Since she was taking Coumadin® (warfarin, a blood thinner), the staff was concerned that this might be a serious problem so they arranged for her to visit her primary care physician. This was a good plan of action except she was dropped off all by herself in the doctor's waiting room, without any paperwork explaining her problem. She certainly was not able to remember why she had been sent! She returned to the ALF a few hours later with prescriptions for antibiotics, cough medicine and a diuretic/water pill. I can only surmise that neither she nor the doctor were able to figure out why she was there. All she knew was that she had a cough and chronic shortness of breath. She was treated for bronchitis and congestive heart failure (CHF) and a chest x-ray (CXR) was ordered.

Whenever there was any medical decision to be made for Aunt Jeanette, Nancy would call me, her brother the doctor, to discuss what had transpired. When she told me about Jeanette's visit to the doctor, I indicated it was baffling since Jeanette was sent solely because her eye was red. But I added that if she had told the doctor that she had shortness of breath and was coughing, then the treatment plan seemed appropriate. I figured Jeanette might have CHF based on her symptoms and that the CXR would help guide her therapy. To our surprise, the CXR revealed a mass in the middle of her chest and a CT scan was suggested. Several days passed before the CT scan results were forwarded to me. They revealed an 8-cm mass in the central region of her chest with a large pleural effusion* (fluid collection) and multiple smaller lesions (masses) in her lungs consistent with metastatic* (disseminated) cancer. Nancy and I had discussed these disturbing results at some length the day before my arrival in South Florida.

I knew what lay ahead. I had to set up a plan and would employ my "begin with the end in mind strategy." First, I had to talk to Mom about Jeanette's test results and what they meant. Next I would communicate with my brother Lewis, and then Jeanette, and lastly with her sister-in-law, Eleanor. The plan was to have an information blitz, rapidly notifying all other family members so that everyone was in the loop as quickly as possible. The plan was set. I would discuss this with Jeanette at one o'clock Sunday afternoon when my medical conference concluded.

We arrived at Aunt Jeanette's assisted living facility with an entourage that included my sister Nancy and her partner, Clare, along with my mother and her dog, Benji. (This would be the first time I discussed bad news with a pet in the room). As we entered her room, we found my Aunt Jeanette in her sweltering apartment, sitting in her recliner. There was a book nearby but it was not opened. Neither the radio nor TV was on. She said she was waiting for her lunch to be delivered.

"Hi, *DAVID*", Jeanette exclaimed as she opened the door to her apartment. "It is so nice to see you, When did you get in town?"

"I arrived last night," I responded, "and I am attending a medical conference this weekend. I also came to see Mom, Nancy, and you."

"Come on in," she said opening the door widely, "this is where I live now. It's a building with a lot of old people," she laughed. "Have you seen my new place before?" (I had been to this apartment at least 10 times) "Sit down and relax a bit. Can I get you something cold to drink?"

"This is a very nice place Aunt Jeanette," I responded "and I have been here before, most recently about four months ago when I was in town for Mom's birthday party."

"Oh, that's right," she said scratching her head, "everybody was in town for that event. Tell me about your boys, what are they up to these days?"

"Both boys are in college and working toward graduation, I hope," I told her.

"Well, I don't have to tell you how hard jobs are to come by these days, but I am sure your boys will be successful if they take after you," she remarked kindly.

We talked about her plants, which seemed a bit wilted. She was not watering them. My mom asked Jeanette, "Do you remember how far we had to walk to school? Why did Mom and Pop live so far away from our school?"

Jeanette replied, "We lived there to be close to where Pop worked and it was close to our cousins. Don't you remember? You know that those cousins lived to be nearly 100 years old."

Mom said, "We do come from a family of people who live a long time."

Jeanette responded, "I know I'm living on borrowed time. I just turned 90 and that's how old Mom and Pop were when they died." It was at that moment that Mom thought it was an opportune time for me to tell Aunt Jeanette about her condition and interjected, "Jeanette, what a coincidence, that's one of the reasons why David is here today."

I gave Mom a stare as if to say we could have been a bit more delicate. I took a deep breath and said, "Aunt Jeanette, Mom is referring to the tests you had recently and I would like to discuss the results with you." She acknowledged, saying, "I remembered the tests." I proceeded to tell her about the fluid in her chest and the mass in her lung. She nodded her head that she understood. There was a disappointed look on her face, almost as if to say, "*I expected something like this but thought I could have avoided it.*" I quickly told her that there would be no kind of therapy for this condition. She slowly admitted, "I wouldn't want any even if some were available. I just want you to assure me that if I have any pain it can be controlled."

"Aunt Jeanette, since you did not have much pain after your hysterectomy or your fractured hip, I feel confident that you will not have much pain from this either." I added that Hospice could be consulted and they would be able to treat her in her apartment, make her comfortable and help with management of any pain while helping her maintain her dignity. This information seemed to put her at ease.

As quickly as I had initiated my discussion, Jeanette changed the subject, asking, "How much longer will you be staying and when do you expect to return to south Florida to visit me again?"

"I will be leaving this afternoon," I replied, "and I am not sure exactly when I will return, probably in 4 to 5 weeks." We took this as our clue that Jeanette was tiring and wanted some time to be alone, so we prepared to leave. We all gave Aunt Jeanette big hugs, and Nancy, Clare, and Mom told her they would return in a few days. At that point, her lunch arrived and we bid farewell.

After our visit, I drove alone to visit with my Aunt Eleanor, Jeanette's 90 year old sister-in-law. They had known each other since the fourth grade, long before they became related by marriage. She was not aware that any testing had been done on Jeanette, and I knew she would be surprised and upset about the information I would give her.

Since I had called before my arrival, I found Aunt Eleanor waiting for me at the end of a long hallway on the fourth floor of her Independent Living Facility building. As she invited me into her apartment, I noticed how neat, tidy, and elegant it was. Most of the artwork that I had grown up seeing in her home was hanging on the walls, lending a familiar and comforting surrounding for her and for me.

"David," she said greeting me with a big hug. "How nice of you to visit me today. What brings you to south Florida? Please, sit down and let me get you a cold drink." I sat down, enjoyed a sip of iced tea, and nervously grabbed a handful of nuts from a bowl on an end table.

"I came to visit Mom, Nancy, Clare, Aunt Jeanette, and you. I have also been attending an educational program in Fort Lauderdale," I responded.

"How are Chad and Jake?" she inquired. I proceeded to fill her in on the details of their college experiences. "How have you been Aunt Eleanor? How are my cousins and all your grandchildren and great grandchildren?" My aunt ran down the list of who was doing what in her family and as usual, I was impressed with their accomplishments.

As I had walked through the lobby of her building on my way to Eleanor's apartment, I noticed a large number of walkers and wheel chairs parked outside the dining room. This indicated to me that the residents in her facility were frail and aged. Aunt Eleanor acknowledged, "Many of my friends have been ill or died. There has been quite a bit of turnover in my community." That did not take me by surprise and it provided an opening to transition to the purpose of my visit.

I jumped at the opening and proceeded to review with her the status of Aunt Jeanette's health. She reacted with sadness, disappointment and, I sensed, embarrassment. Much like Aunt Jeanette, there was an understanding that we all die one day but we never consider the circumstances beforehand. As I finished my iced tea, I asked Eleanor to pass the information along to her children, my cousins, and to give them all my regards. As I left her apartment, I gave her a big hug and noticed how small and frail she had become. I walked to my car with a sense of accomplishment and relief.

In addition, I reflected on the impact my two aunts had had on my life. Both were well-educated (Eleanor was a high school English teacher) and well-traveled, providing an influence that encouraged curiosity and propelling me to excel in my education and life.

Driving to meet up with my sister and Mom gave me some time to clear my head from the events of the day. No nephew would ever want to have this type of conversation with beloved aunts, but I realized based on the experiences I have had in my career, I would not consider anyone more capable for the job than I was. I really did consider it part of my duty to my family to take on this task. As I was the family member with the medical experience, my sister Nancy had become Aunt Jeanette's health care surrogate and was saddled with the responsibility of day-to-day management and coordination of her care. Nancy contacted the staff of the ALF and requested that Jeanette remain in the facility until she died. The ALF administration was gracious and, because of Jeanette's pleasant nature, they agreed. Hospice was contacted and Jeanette was enrolled. This was a bit tricky because with her diminished short term memory, we were not certain that she would be able to understand and give her consent.

Although I discussed Hospice care in an earlier chapter about my father, I feel compelled to share some additional thoughts. In the years I have been in practice I have had the occasion to learn a great deal about our local organization and the national Hospice and palliative care movement. Most people associate Hospice with cancer deaths and then, only in the dying stage. Nothing could be further from the truth. Hospice is an organization dedicated to care for patients who are dying, and for providing palliative (comfort care). This means that any person with a terminal diagnosis (one that can lead to death) is eligible to enroll. This includes end-stage congestive heart failure and end-stage Alzheimer's disease to name a few. Insurance companies allow patients to take advantage of Hospice and Medicare through federal government funding, even encouraging enrollment in Hospice. In fact, in the county in which I practice, up to 45 percent of Medicare enrollees die while under the care of Hospice. The rationale is that it helps relieve some of the discomfort of the patients and their family members. With this in mind, it was clear that Hospice care was a very good fit for Aunt Jeanette as she had a terminal diagnosis of Alzheimer's disease *and* cancer.

Within a short period of time, it was apparent that Jeanette required additional daily attention. Nancy arranged for 8 hours of daily care to be provided by private aides. Since similar needs arose when Dad was ill, Nancy contracted with the same private duty aides who had taken care of him. What started out as 8 hour shifts gradually evolved into 16 and eventually 24 hours a day, 7 days a week. Jeanette was not able to do any of her own care. She could not even leave her room to go for her meals. Jeanette had become urine incontinent and was even showing her stubborn side by not cooperating with the aides when she needed bathing. As the cancer progressed, eventually filling her lungs with tumors and fluid, breathing became more and more difficult. There was a benefit from having oxygen provided, but she did not always find it comfortable to use.

In her last months, Jeanette's visitors included only close family, her aides, and the staff member who worked at her facility. Nancy and Clare did the bulk of the visiting. Mom seemed to lack the patience, especially with regard to Jeanette's refusal to bathe. It was difficult for Mom to see her treasured sister, the last living member of her immediate family, dying. I spoke to Nancy regularly, getting updates and answering her questions about what to do and what to expect. Within the past year Nancy had dealt with our father's illness and death and now was in the middle of the same thing with Aunt Jeanette. Nancy had been a manager at a CVS store, a job that required a 60 to 70 hour work week. She was now consumed with dealing with the dying process of our much loved Aunt. Nancy, like her brothers, learned lessons from our father who had told all his children, "*You put your head down and charge forward. Nothing is too difficult for a Bernstein.*"

Aunt Jeanette continued to deteriorate, but suddenly she rallied. She asked her aides to get her out of bed and dress her. She spoke to several family members on the phone and spent quality time with my mother and her sister-in-law Eleanor. She told Eleanor that she had been a wonderful friend and sister-in-law. Jeanette then turned her attention to her bird and went back to her room. My mother, sister and Clare also had an opportunity to spend time with Jeanette on the day that she showed a sudden burst of energy. The following day she lapsed into profound fatigue. Day by day she became weaker and weaker, eventually dying within a week of that special day she rallied. Her death was peaceful and occurred in her sleep.

The call from my sister informing me of Aunt Jeanette's passing came while I was ending my vacation in Key West, Florida. Since it was just a four hour drive to the funeral home, I was able to make changes to my plans.

My observations about the funeral for a 91 year old are that at this age, one has out lived most if not all of their friends and many relatives. Therefore there are very few people alive or healthy enough to attend. Those who are able to be there know that the deceased has lived a long and full life, and in most cases their suffering has ended. This should limit the degree of sadness at the funeral. I found one aspect of Aunt Jeanette's funeral somewhat amusing to me. The Rabbi assigned by the funeral home to perform the service had never met Jeanette. Thirty minutes before the graveside burial he gathered the family and asked us to tell him a little bit about her. Eight family members sat around a large table and each spoke briefly. Aunt Eleanor started, "Jeanette loved her family and enjoyed spending time with each of us." My brother Lewis added, "She loved music, was always singing, and enjoyed going to Broadway shows. She even saved all her Playbills. She sang in choirs and criticized bad voices. She was independent, always on the go, feisty and stubborn." Mom said," She was a loving daughter and sister, and I was always able to count on her. She had many friends and she enjoyed traveling with them." My cousin Jeff recalled stories about when she used to babysit for him and his brother and sister. I recalled that she loved her job and from what she always told me, was probably smarter than her bosses. She made great pancakes.

One half hour later at the funeral, in elegant words as only a Rabbi could do, he told us how Jeanette loved music and theater, loved to sing and criticized bad voices. She was always on the go, and loved her family and enjoyed babysitting for her nieces and nephews who loved her homemade pancakes. Sitting listening to these words were the same family members who had sat with the Rabbi. Three of Nancy's friends and four of Aunt Jeanette's aides made up the remainder of those participating in the funeral. Tears were shed although we all knew that Aunt Jeanette did lead a happy and full life, and at the end, her death was a peaceful one.

Notes on living longer:

- Alzheimer's disease robs individuals of short term memories, but most often an individual can maintain long term memories. Under the right circumstances and with family connections and personality, independence can be maintained.
- With advancing age, patients with Alzheimer's disease are at risk for multiple conditions associated with age such as heart disease, cancer, and complications associated with falls.
- Strong family connections will enable the potential of higher level of support and ultimately a more pleasant aging process.
- A family member, acting as a representative/health care surrogate, can be extremely valuable in navigating the waters of today's healthcare environment.
- Here are 5 key considerations for making this process smoother:
  - ✓ Be connected throughout life.
  - ✓ When you are with family and friends, be present and engaged.
  - ✓ Maintain strong relationships with family, friends, and community groups.
  - ✓ Promote spirituality in your life each and every day.
  - ✓ Have a well thought-out Advance Directive and assign a Health Care Surrogate(s) who can represent your views/ideas/wishes in the event you become incapacitated.

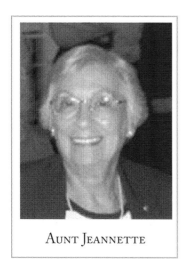

AUNT JEANNETTE

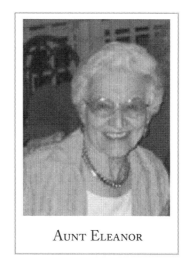

AUNT ELEANOR

Resources and Links:

Alzheimer's Foundation of America, Caring for Persons, one at a time. *www.alzfdn.org/*

www.Helpguide.org
Recommended Articles:

- Alzheimer's Disease
- Dementia
- Caregiving

Isaacson, Richard (2011) *Alzheimer's Treatment; Alzheimer's Prevention*, Miami Beach, Florida, AD Education Consultants, Inc.

Mace, Nancy and Rabins, Peter (1981) *The 36- HOUR DAY* New York, Warner Books

Living GRACEfully

We don't beat the reaper by living longer.
We beat the reaper by living fully.
– Randy Pausch, 2007

A s I reflect on the lessons I have learned during my 30 years as a practicing physician, I realize how much I have absorbed from both within and beyond the walls of my office. These lessons have not been limited to medicine per se; what I've really been learning is how to live a long and fulfilling life.

My "Aunt" Eleanor (not a blood relative of mine), whom I mention in the story about Aunt Jeanette, has shown me much about living a **GRACE**ful life.

She always had a **Goal,** which was to help make those around her be the best they could be. As a high school English teacher she taught the finest literature allowed in public schools and always demanded excellence from her students. I know this because I used to watch her correct term papers and I had the pleasure of discussing several books with her. She was demanding, and neither her students nor I could get away with any nonsense. She saw to it that her own children got excellent educations, too, and "made something" of themselves. In retirement, she turned her attention to her husband and set goals for traveling and enjoying their new leisure. When he developed Alzheimer's disease, she worked to make his life the best and safest possible.

She had excellent **Roots.** I had met her parents, and could see they had been good role models; they lived well into their eighties. Aunt Eleanor followed their example, made appropriate adjustments to her diet and activities and lived into her nineties.

The elders in my family, including Aunt Eleanor, all lived through the depression and their experiences helped to shape their **Attitudes.** They all believed that getting ahead in life had to do with perseverance. She emulated this and taught it to her children, nieces, nephews, grandchildren and students. Nothing was unattainable if you tried. She applied this in her own life as well: even though she was a great cook, her attempts at Matzo balls never turned out well (they were always heavy and dense—not the way they should be) but she kept at it. Her attitude was amazing, even if her Matzo balls were not!

Aunt Eleanor had **Companionship.** She maintained her connections to family and friends throughout her life. I still remember, way back in my childhood, how she would talk about some of her closest friends. She was still lovingly talking about them the last time I spoke with her—when she was 91. She maintained close bonds with her children and excelled in connecting with her grandchild. She knew and remembered every aspect of their lives. As she got older, despite her poor hearing, she managed to understand, and remember the small details of any project any one of us was doing. While I was writing this book, she never failed to ask about it each time I saw her. I was touched by how well she remembered specific subjects I planned to include.

Since I did not live with my aunt, I cannot give a detailed account about how she interacted with her **Environment.** I do know that she kept her weight under control, visited her doctor and took his advice. When he recommended heart valve replacement in her mid-80s, she agreed; it was done successfully and extended her life by nearly a decade.

During one of my many visits to California I joined my Aunt Flo (who by coincidence was 91 years old, just like my Aunt Eleanor) for a cup of coffee. I told her about my plans to write this book and she wondered out loud if she was going to be in it. On my very next visit she insisted that she deserved a place in my book. (She is a funny lady). She was *not* going to take no for an answer and even asked which chapter she would be in! I politely told her that my book was almost completed and I did not know where I could fit her in. As I considered this Epilogue it became quite apparent that she fit right in and belonged *here*, in my concluding remarks about living **GRACE**fully.

Aunt Flo grew up in Detroit and moved to California after World War II. She settled down with my uncle and raised three children. Like most women in the 1950s and 60s, her **Goal** in life was to raise a happy family and be a supportive wife to her husband. She excelled in those roles and achieved her goals. It is important to acknowledge this: just *having* the goal is what counts, not whether society thinks it has virtue. Her other ambition was to nurture her artistic side. Well into her late 80s, she worked with pottery and other crafts, getting great enjoyments out of it.

Aunt Flo's **Roots** are unknown to me but since she lived into her 90s, I can say that along with choosing the right parents, she must have recognized the effect diet and exercise have on longevity, not to mention quality of life.

Flo had an **Attitude** about age; it didn't matter how old a person was, she accepted all ages into her book club and other groups to which she belonged. This attitude paid off for her: at 91 she was the oldest member of her book club and the only one who wasn't required to use email to communicate with the other book club members. They gave her a "pass"—she had earned it!

Aunt Flo set standards for **Companionship**. She had a loving and supporting relationship with her husband, *whom I am certain might not have been the easiest person to live with*. She worked hard to keep immediate and distant family connected. She has been, in part, responsible for her side of the family trekking to family get-togethers on the East Coast, and for putting together great family events when we traveled to the West Coast. She stayed in close touch with all her grandchildren and made it a point to know the details of their lives as they grew up. At the ripe age of 91, I saw her walk down the aisle of her granddaughter's wedding and "kvell" (a Yiddish word meaning beam with pride) at the sight of the beautiful bride. At the party that followed, I marveled as she was surrounded by friends, some of whom went back 60 and 70 years. It was a treat for me to sit with this lively crew of active, loving, senior adults.

In addition to my family, I have had the pleasure for over two decades of taking care of a special group of aging adults: my retired Salvation Army officers. As a group they are wonderful—caring, respectful, loyal, and tightly connected to one another. Once I had demonstrated my skills and temperament to my first patient from the group, many of the others flocked to my office. I have to give a lot of kudos to my office staff, especially my office manager, Vicki, who presented the nurturing side of my practice. She performed her job in a way that exceeded the expectation of all my patients, especially the retired Salvation Army officers. Within a year of the first officer becoming a patient of mine, I must have had 30 or 40! I felt like the manager of a sports team who got 40 number-one draft picks all at once. Each patient expressed his or her gratitude at the end of the office visit and sometimes thanked me for taking such good care of their band of friends. In return, I have expressed *my* gratitude to them for being such exemplary patients. As a group, they have had a hugely positive impact on my practice and have helped fuel my personal growth as well.

Jim and Ruth stand out within this group and within my entire practice, actually, for their complete embodiment of **GRACE**. They are my "poster children" for how to live life with **GRACE**. Because they are so modest, I must not have understood their position among the other retired officers at the time of their first visit. It eventually became clear to me that they had been at the pinnacle of the Salvation Army leadership hierarchy. Jim had run the organization for the entire USA!

As a couple, Jim and Ruth have been inseparable. From what I've observed, the quality of their lives is based upon the fact that they *live their lives in tandem*. Their lives have been dedicated to service to their church and mankind. They have been involved in service to others, one way or another, all their lives. Their **Goal and Purpose** has been to make a difference for their fellow man.

I met them when they were in their early 70s and hardly showed signs of slowing down. In a four year period of time, they were called back into service three times and did not hesitate to accept each assignment. As a team, they were sent from Florida to the state of Washington to run the largest center in the State after an abrupt vacancy. Imagine a man and woman in their early 80s responsible for the organization in the largest region within the State of Oregon. They returned home in time to check in with their doctor (me) and then came the next assignment: filling in for the regional director in Chattanooga, Tennessee for six months until a replacement could be found. After a brief hiatus, which included another visit to their doctor (me, again), they were sent to Johnson City Tennessee to substitute for the regional director who had become ill. After each assignment, I would inquire," *Why?*" They would just look at me, tilt their heads to the side and say, "Why not? We are good at it, we love it, and they love us. Isn't that why you do what you do, Doctor? It gives us a **Goal** to accomplish." I could hardly argue with them; it kept them engaged, active and alive.

Ruth regarded her **Roots** or genes as excellent; her parents lived into their 80s, but Jim's roots were the opposite. His parents had died fairly early in life and left him genes that lead to high blood pressure, diabetes, high cholesterol and coronary artery disease. By the time I became his physician, he had already had a coronary artery bypass (open heart surgery). When I assumed his care after he moved to Florida, he told me, "I am in your hands Doctor; I will do whatever you tell me." He was not kidding; he took every medication I prescribed, ate exceptionally well and walked at 5:30 every morning, "rain or shine." Even when they were out of town on assignment, Jim and Ruth complied with my instructions. They would go to a local hospital lab and have their blood drawn for the tests I ordered so I could remain up to date with their care. These instructions were followed on time and without objections. I characterize Jim's behavior as the best way to deal with the bad **Roots** and Ruth's as being unbelievably supportive.

Jim and Ruth live their lives with an **Attitude** of optimism, love for their fellow man and gratitude. Their altruism knows no bounds and anyone who interacts with them sees it immediately.

Jim and Ruth are inseparable **Companions**. They look at each other the same way they must have on their honeymoon. During one of our office visits, I acted devilishly and attempted to get them to disagree on something. They saw right through my ruse. Ruth said, "I know what you're up to and I am too smart to fall for that trick." I just smiled.

Jim and Ruth have children (I have met their daughter and she is the spitting image of her mother), and they have a large community of extended family in Florida and across the country with whom they stay connected. It's easy to see the love they have for their fellow retired officers; they speak about each other as if they are blood relatives. They are entwined in the lives of others in a way I have never experienced.

As for their **Environment,** and despite what I consider advanced age and multiple chronic medical problems, both wake up before the sun rises and walk for at least one hour before attending to their devotionals, which are then followed by a "healthy" breakfast. Since Jim has diabetes, he and Ruth eat a low-carbohydrate, low-fat diet, and their blood test results validate their adherence. The time spent in their devotionals also can be compared to a meditative or a relaxed period or reflection, another beneficial element to the enhancement of one's health.

I have never had more attentive patients in all my years in practice. Whatever medication I prescribed prompted questions such as, "Why do I need that medicine? What will it do for me? How long will I have to take it? What are the side effects? Are you sure I need it?" but once I answered them thoroughly, they followed my directions to a T. I'm thankful they had the good fortune of seeing the favorable results of their treatments and adherence to them.

The preparation of this book has directed personal reflections of where **GRACE** exists in my life. From as far back as I can remember I have been **Goal**-oriented: getting into college, medical school, and then becoming the best doctor I could be. Now that I am middle-aged, I realize I must prepare for new ventures (or adventures) in my life. My next milestone will be my retirement, which means developing a plan with goals and a purpose, something I think about every day, especially on really difficult ones. I acknowledge the **Roots** I have, and have taken steps to overcome what I view as negative genetic traits. I monitor my cholesterol, blood pressure, and blood sugar as they are reflective of conditions my father dealt with for much of his life. Surprisingly, being a doctor led to sacrifices with regard to my own health. I have learned my lessons, though, and reversed some of those poor decisions.

My **Attitude** has been another of my strong suits, but there is always room for improvement. I have especially learned about the value of *gratitude*. I have led a conservative life in many respects; as a physician and parent I have been reluctant to take risks but as life has evolved, and from lessons learned from my patients, I have learned to be more **Adventurous** and go out on skinny branches. Life has more exhilaration when one stretches outside one's comfort zone. This is not to say I plan to lead a life of risk-taking but I do realize the wisdom in not delaying things for "another day." As life has shown me, sometimes that day never comes.

I have also learned about Companionship from my patients. I have developed concentric circles in my life, starting with my parents and siblings and extending out to more distant relatives. Through relationships within my family, I've learned to understand and provide unconditional love as well as the importance of appreciating and cherishing each other. My precious wife and our children are the grounding force of that love, the foundation for my own goals, roots, attitudes, and companionship. This encourages me to respond to my environment positively, to be my best mentally, physically and spiritually.

Interacting with my **Environment** has taken many roads over the years, but I have always used some form of physical activity as a diversion from life stresses. There were years when my children participated in all sorts of activities that focused my attention away from a regular physical routine for my mind and body. I never lost sight, however, of the need to ensure physical exercise as a component in my life. Over the years, I have become much more cognizant of my other habits, such as sleep (getting enough of it each night!), and have taken steps to reconcile my patterns to enhance my overall health.

What I recommend for my patients and to readers of this book is to find the Jim or Ruth inside you and live life **GRACE**fully. Dissect each element of **GRACE** and incorporate the lessons learned in the lives portrayed in this book and, I assure you, you can enhance the quality and quantity of your life. Greater contentment will follow.

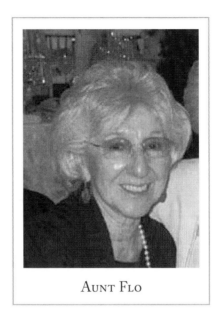

AUNT FLO

Resources and Links:

www.Helpguide.org
Recommended Articles:

- *Healthy Aging Tips*
- *Eating Well*
- *Senior Exercise and Fitness Tips*
- *Emotional Healthy Help*
- *How to Improve Your Memory*

◆ ◆ ◆

Dear Readers,

As the author I am very curious as to how you, my readers will tackle GRACE. Please contact me through my website: www. davidbernsteinmd.com and share with me what YOU'RE doing to live your life with GRACE…

If you are on Facebook, "follow-me" at www.facebook.com/ davidbernsteinmd for interesting blogs and updates on aging GRACEfully.

Now I would like to as for a "small" favor. Could you please take a minute or two to leave a Review on Amazon using this link: http://amzn.to/1A2o1tE.

This feedback will help me to continue to write the kind of books like this to help people.

To a long and healthy life,
David Bernstein, MD

Glossary

AAA—Abdominal aortic aneurysm

The aorta is the main blood vessel that carries blood away from the heart to the rest of the body. An aneurysm is an abnormal enlargement in the wall of a blood vessel. An abdominal aortic aneurysm, therefore, is an abnormal enlargement of the lower part of the aorta as it extends through the abdominal area. The aorta is an elastic blood vessel, filled with blood that's under pressure as it is pumped from the heart. Aneurysms can develop in weakened segments of the blood vessel wall, distending it like a balloon. When I describe aneurysms to my patients, I tell them it is like a bubble in a garden hose.

The major predisposing factors contributing to the development of an aneurysm are smoking, family history, congenital defects, injury, infection, and high blood pressure. Each year in the U.S., abdominal aortic aneurysms cause 15,000 deaths. The majority of these deaths are due to the sudden rupture of the aneurysm and rapid internal bleeding. Aneurysms can be diagnosed with a physical exam (by palpation), and by routine radiological tests such as X-rays, CT scans and MRI. Sometimes they are detected as what's called an "incidental finding" on one of these radiological tests. A study performed in the 1960's revealed that the risk of rupture was directly related to the size of the aneurysm—the larger the aneurysm, the greater the risk. This was the knowledge base available to me when I was treating Mel. The treatment at that time was to send these patients (who by nature of the condition were old), through a major abdominal operation to replace the dilated aortic, to prevent its rupture and the patient's certain death.

Anemia—see chapter 8

CT scan

Computerized (or computed) tomography, and often formerly referred to as computerized axial tomography (CAT) scan, is an X-ray procedure that combines many X-ray images with the aid of a computer to generate cross-sectional views and, if needed, three-dimensional images of the internal organs and structures of the body. Computerized tomography is more commonly known by its abbreviated names, CT scan or CAT scan. A CT scan is used to define normal and abnormal structures in the body and/or assist in procedures by helping to accurately guide the placement of instruments or treatments.

Coronary Artery Bypass surgery

CABG surgery is performed on individuals with coronary artery disease who have severe obstruction to the vessels that supply blood to the heart. A Thoracic (chest) surgeon also known as a Heart surgeon creates new routes around narrowed and blocked arteries, allowing sufficient blood flow to deliver oxygen and nutrients to the heart muscle.

Leaky Mitral Valve

Chronic mitral valve regurgitation, the most common type, develops slowly. Many people with this problem have a valve that is prone to wear and tear. As the person gets older, the valve gets weak and no longer closes tightly. Other causes include heart failure, rheumatic fever, congenital heart disease, a calcium buildup in the valve, and other cardiac problems.

Acute mitral valve regurgitation develops quickly and can be life-threatening. It happens when the valve or nearby tissue ruptures suddenly. Instead of a slow leak, blood builds up quickly in the left side of the heart. The heart doesn't have time to adjust to this sudden buildup of blood the way it does with the slow buildup of blood in chronic regurgitation. Common causes of acute regurgitation are heart attack, a heart infection called endocarditis, or a sudden rupture of one of the muscles that hold it in place.

Lung Cancer

Primary lung cancer forms in the lung tissue, usually in the cells lining air passages. The two main types of cancers, small cell lung cancer and non-small cell lung cancers, are diagnosed based the appearance of cells under a microscope. Most lung cancers are non-small cell type and these are further subcategorized. Sometimes, people will have cancer from another part of their body travel or metastasize to their lungs. This is called secondary lung cancer, because the lungs are secondary compared to the original, primary location of the cancer. Secondary lung cancer is not lung cancer but rather the type of cancer from its original site such as breast or colon cancer. Such cancers are treated differently than primary lung cancers because it's a different disease.

When a lung cancer is diagnosed, the pathologist assigns it a type (either non-small cell lung cancer or small cell lung cancer) and then assigns a stage to the cancer. The stage is a formal classification that signifies the extent of the cancer and determines the treatment offered to the patient. Lower stage numbers signify less advanced cancers; for example, a stage I is an early-stage cancer and most likely will have not spread from its original place of origin. The stage IV cancer indicates an advanced stage cancer and may appear in the lung as well as other areas of the body (metastases).

Lung cancer is one of the most common cancers. In 2007, lung cancer accounted for approximately 15 percent of all cancer diagnoses yet 28 percent of all cancer deaths. It is the second most diagnosed cancer in men and women (after prostate for men and breast cancer for women). *It is the number one cause of death from cancer each year in both men and women.* Because lung cancer can take years to develop, it is mostly found in older people—as a matter of fact, the average age of a person diagnosed with lung cancer is 71. Overall, lung cancer affects men more than women, but the gap is closing. It is well recognized that cigarette smoking is the cause of most lung cancers but there are other risk factors. Exposure to asbestos, radon, environmental toxins and secondhand smoke can cause lung cancer as well.

Metastasis

Metastasis is the process by which cancer spreads from the place at which it first arose as a primary tumor to distant locations in the body. Metastasis depends on the cancer cells acquiring two separate abilities – increased motility and invasiveness. Cells that metastasize are basically of the same kind as those in the original tumor. If a cancer arises in the lung and metastasizes to the liver, the cancer cells in the liver are lung cancer cells. However, the cells have acquired increased motility and the ability to invade another organ.

Pleural effusion

A pleural effusion is a collection of fluid in the space between the two linings (pleura) of the lung.

When we breathe, it is like a bellows. We inhale air into our lungs and the ribs move out and the diaphragm moves down. For the lung to expand, its lining has to slide along with the chest wall movement. For this to happen, both the lungs and the ribs are covered with a slippery lining called the pleura. A small amount of fluid acts as a lubricant for these two surfaces to slide easily against each other.

Too much fluid impairs the ability of the lung to expand and move. A pleural effusion is not normal. It is not a disease but rather a complication of an underlying illness. Extra fluid (effusion) can occur for a variety of reasons. Common classification systems divide pleural effusions based on the chemistry composition of the fluid and what causes the effusion to be formed.

Shingles/ Post herpetic neuralgia

Shingles (herpes zoster) is a painful, blistering skin rash due to the varicella-zoster virus, the virus that causes chickenpox.

After contracting chickenpox, the virus remains inactive (becomes dormant) in certain nerves in the body. Shingles occurs after the virus becomes active again in these nerves years later. The reason the virus suddenly becomes active again it 7is not clear. Often only one attack occurs. Shingles may develop in any age group, but it more likely to occur during one for the following circumstances: individuals over age 60, exposure to chickenpox before age 1 or when the immune system is weakened by medications or disease.

If an adult or child has direct contact with the shingles rash and did not have chickenpox as a child or a chickenpox vaccine, they can develop chickenpox, not shingles. The first symptom is usually one-sided pain, tingling, or burning. The pain and burning may be severe and is usually present before any rash appears. Red patches on the skin, followed by small fluid filled blisters, form in most people. Health care provider can make the diagnosis by looking at the rash and reviewing the medical history. Tests are rarely needed for confirmation.

Health care providers may prescribe a medicine that fights the virus, called an antiviral drug. This drug helps reduce pain, prevent complications, and shorten the course of the disease when administered shortly after the onset of the blisters Herpes zoster usually clears up in 2 to 3 weeks and rarely returns.

Persistent pain in the area where the shingles occurred may last from months to years and is referred to as post herpetic neuralgia.

Post herpetic neuralgia is more likely to occur in people over age 60. It occurs when the nerves have been damaged after an outbreak of shingles. Pain ranges from mild to very severe.

A herpes zoster vaccine is available. Older adults who receive the herpes zoster vaccine are less likely to have complications from shingles. The United States Advisory Committee on Immunization Practices (ACIP) has recommended that adults older than 60 receive the herpes zoster vaccine as part of routine medical care.

Spinal Stenosis—see chapter 8

Stents (Cardiac)

Stents are devices placed into an artery (such as a coronary artery) to keep the vessel open and they have been used in lieu of balloon angioplasty to treat patients with coronary artery disease (CAD) for the past 15-20 years,. They are used because of their better long term outcomes of keeping coronary open longer than angioplasty alone.

Ulcer Disease—chapter 8

References

Chapter 1
Why I Practice Medicine Introduction

Geriatrics, retrieved December 22, 2011 from Wikipedia, the free encyclopedia en.wikipedia.org/wiki/Geriatrics

Wilders, E. (2011) *Want Job Satisfaction? Not helpful? You can block en.wikipedia.org results when you're signed in to search.en.wikipedia.org Choose Geriatrics,* Medscape News Student, and Retrieved June 2011 from http://www.medscape.com/viewarticle/7376179997

Chapter 2
GRACE

Pasternak, Harley with Bolt, Ethan (2005); 5 Factor Fitness: The Diet and Fitness Secret of Hollywood's A-List New York,NY Penguin Group (USA) Incorporated

Connelly, A. Scott & Coleman, Carol (2003) Body Rx: Dr. Scott Connelly's 6-Pack Prescription, New York, Berkeley Publishing Company 2003

Chapter 3
Working into Old Age

Rowan, Roy (2011), *Never Too Late: A 90-Year-Old's Pursuit of a Whirlwind Life*, Globe Pequot Press, 4/1/2011 *hardcover*, Lyons Press, 2012 *paperback*,

Chapter 4
100th Birthdays

K8 N (2009,October) *Centenarian-Secrets.* Retrieved October 3, 2011from
http://k8n.hubpages.com/hub/Centenarian-Secrets

NY Times (2010, October) Park, Alice *Secrets of the Centenarians, Life Before, During and After 100.* Retrieved August 27, 2012 from
http://www.nytimes.com/interactive/2010/10/19/health/20101018-centenarians-voices-photos.html

Sho H. History and characteristics of Okinawan longevity food. Asia Pac J Clin Nutr. 2001; 10: 159–164.

Chapter 5
Birth Certificates //Gratitude

Keogh, Justin WL, Kilding, Andrew, Pidgon,Phillippa, Ashley, Linda & Gillis, Dawn, *Physical Benefits of Dancing for Healthy Older Adults: A Review* Journal on Aging and Physical Activity (2009), 17, pp 470-500

Kushner, Harold S. (1996) *How Good Do We Have to Be?* Boston, Little Brown & Co.

Levy, Becca (2012) *Positive Attitude - Healthy Aging for Women Baby Boomers.* Retrieved August 27, 2012 from www.healthy-aging-for-women-babyboomers.com/positive-attitude...

ScienceDaily (2009) *Dance Your Way to Successful Aging.* Retrieved February 19, 2012 from
http://sciencedaily.com/releases/2009/04/090401103127.htm

Weil, Andrew (2007) *Bad Attitude Toward Aging?* Retrieved October 2011 from DrWeil.com Q & A library at http://www.drweil.com/drw/u/QAA400281/bad-attitude-toward-aging

Chapter 6
Sex, Denial and Home Health Aides

Chapter 7
Environment

American College of Sports Medicine. 2006. *ACSM's Guidelines for Exercise Testing and Prescription* (7th ed.). Philadelphia: Lippincott Williams & Wilkins.

Appel, Lawrence J *Circulation. 2008; 118: 214-215*

Janet, Peter (2012) *50+:Live Better, Long, Eating for Longevity.* Retreived May 29, 2012 from www.webmd.com/healthy-aging/features/eating-longevity?page=3

Gonzales-Wallace, Michael(2010).*Super Body Super Brain.* New York, NY HarperCollins Publishers

Heidemann C, Schulze MB, Franco OH, van Dam RM, Mantzoros CS, Hu FB. Dietary patterns and risk of mortality from cardiovascular disease, cancer, and all causes in a prospective cohort of women. Circulation. 2008; 118; 230–237.

Hyman, Mark (2006) *Ultra-Metabolism.* New York, Scribner

Kravitz, Len (2007) The *25 Most Significant Health Benefits of Physical Activity and Exercise* IDEA Fitness Journal, Volume 4, Number 9

Marcell, T.J. 2003. Sarcopenia: Causes, consequences, and preventions. *Journal of Gerontology, 58A* (10), 911–16.

Pasternak, Harley (2009) *The 5 Factor Diet.* New York, Ballantine Books, an imprint of The Random House Publishing Group.

Sho H. History and characteristics of Okinawan longevity food. Asia Pac J Clin Nutr. 2001; 10: 159–164.

Van Dusen, Allison (2008) *Top Diet Tips As You Age.* Retrieved February 10, 2012 from www.forbes.com

Ward, Elizabeth (2008)Longevity Diet: Healthy Anti-aging Foods, Retrieved November 6, 2011 from www.webmd.com/**diet**/guide/**aging**-well-eating-right-for-longevity

Not helpful? You can block **www.safeaging.org** results when you're signed in to search.www.safeaging.org

Chapter 8
Begin with the End in Mind

Covey, Stephen (1989) *The 7 Habits of Highly Effective People*, New York, Simon and Schuster p 95-144

Groopman, Jerome (2007) *How Doctors Think*. Boston, A Mariner Book, Houghton Mifflin Co.

Newman, David H. (2008) *Hippocrates' Shadow*. New York, Scribner

The Adult Treatment Panel III (ATP III) of the National Cholesterol Education Program– an evidence-based set of guidelines on cholesterol management in 2001 (Executive Summary published in JAMA, 2001;285:2486-2497).

Anemia

http://www.nhlbi.nih.gov/health/health-topics/topics/anemia/

Lung Cancer

www.lungcancer.org

Spinal stenosis

www.spinalstenosis.com

www.Mayoclinic.com

www.niams.gov

Chapter 9
But Doctor, I Am a Good Driver

Alzheimer's Association, *Driving and Dementia*, Alz.org, Driving and Dementia Resource Center Retrieved November 16, 2011 from http://www.alz.org/care/alzheimers-dementia-and-driving.asp

Alzheimer's Association National Board of Directors, approved September 2011, *Driving and Dementia* Retrieved December15, 2011 from http://www.alz.org/documents_custom/statements/driving_and_dementia.pdf

The Hartford Group, *Dementia and Driving: Understanding Dementia and Driving*
http://www.thehartford.com/advance50/dementia-driving

Chapter 10
Dad ~Hospice

NIA.NIH.gov. (2011) *Talking to Your Doctor: A Guide for Older People*. Retrieved January 2, 2012 from http://www.nia.nih.gov/health/publication/talking-your-doctor-guide-older-people/getting-started-choosing-doctor-you-can

ElderparentHelp.com, *Selecting a Doctor*. Retrieved January 2, 2012 from www.elderparenthelp.com/healthcare/selecting-a-doctor

Hospice Foundation of America, http://www.hospicefoundation.org

Suncoast Hospice, www.thehospice.org/

Chapter 11
Aunt Jeanette

NIH: National Institute on Aging (2010) *Home Safety for People with Alzheimer's Disease*, Retrieved November 16, 2011 from http://www.nia.nih.gov/alzheimers/publication/home-safety-people-alzheimers-disease

Healthy Brain Initiative, A National Public Health Road Map to Maintaining Cognitive Health. Retrieved August 30, 2012 from the

Alzheimer's Association http://www.alz.org/national/documents/ report_healthybraininitiative.pdf

Alzheimer's Association, *Brain Health*, Retrieved November 16, 2011from Alz.org/We Can Help, http://www.alz.org/we_can_help_ brain_health_maintain_your_brain.asp

Alzheimer's Association, 2012 *Alzheimer's disease facts and figures.* Alzheimer's and Dementia: The Journal of Alzheimer's Association, March 2012, 8:131-168

Isaacson, Richard (2011) *Alzheimer's Treatment; Alzheimer's Prevention*, Miami Beach, Florida, AD Education Consultants, Inc.

Moseley, Lorimer (2011, Jan 3) Bodymind.org, *Keeping your Brain Active in Old Age*, Retrieved October, 2011 from http://Bodymind. org//novelty-exercise-and-diet-the-cornerstones-of-neural-and-cognitive-plasticity/

Epilogue
Glossary

http://www.sts.org/patient-information/aneurysm-surgery/aortic-aneurysms. retrieved 6/12/2012

http://www.medicinenet.com/cat_scan/article.htm, retrieved 9/2/2012

http://www.medicinenet.com/coronary_artery_bypass_graft/article. htm#1whatis, retrieved 9/22/2012

http://www.medterms.com/script/main/art.asp?articlekey=4407, retrieved 6/12/2012

www.lungcancer.org, retrieved 2/2/2011

http://www.medterms.com/script/main/art.asp?articlekey=4363.
retrieved 9/1/2012

http://www.medicinenet.com/pleural_effusion/article.htm, retrieved
8/17/2012

http://www.nlm.nih.gov/medlineplus/ency/patientinstructions/
000560.htm, retrieved 8/22/2012

http://www.medicinenet.com/script/main/art.asp?articlekey=78804,
retrieved 9/22/2012

Acknowledgments

I give an abundance of credit to my family—Mom, Dad, Lewis and Nancy—for the profound influence they have had on me and my development as a person. Their undying love and encouragement sustains me.

Mom once pointed out to me how frustrated she was with the medical care provided to her mother and father (my grandparents). The realities that surrounded this comment propelled me toward my career in geriatric medicine. Mom and Dad's philosophical wisdom helped shape me and, in turn, this book. I learned from my father to set examples and to strive to accomplish goals.

A driving force for this entire process has been my children, Chad and Jake, who encouraged me along the way with love and support. In the latter efforts of this project my step-children, Russell and Jillian, provided moral support and valuable media advice.

My wife, Melissa, has been the behind-the-scenes editor and the one who challenged me to probe deeper and explore concepts and my feelings about all the subjects in this book. I deeply appreciate her love and the caring manner in which she encourages me.

My extended family, some of whom are mentioned in this book have influenced my development and provided encouragement as I pursued my goal of bringing this book to fruition.

My patients, who for 30 years have allowed me to develop as a person and a physician and given me countless subjects to ponder. They have provided me with reasons to laugh and to cry. I single out Barbra Johnston for her assistance with editorial suggestions.

I have had many mentors in both my personal and professional life, too numerous to mention them all by name but they include teachers in public school as well as college and medical school professors who shaped how I think. Dr. Bruce Robinson while a professor at the University of South Florida residency program was particularly influential in my choosing a career in geriatric medicine.

My friend Tim McGivern and a group of men I got to know through him gave me balance and support to get though difficult times and allowed me to reflect in ways that clarified my thought process.

It would have been impossible to succeed without the support of many professional friends and those who stand out are Stanton Tripodis who has cross covered for me on weekends and holidays for over 20 years and my great friend Jim Fischer who has always been there for me from our days as interns together until the present day, many thanks.

Martha Murphy, my book coach for this entire process, believed in this project from the start. Among other things, she nailed the title for my book, capturing the bittersweet nature of aging in a way that also reflects my sense of humor. I know without her there would be no words on the paper. Additionally, Jane Aronoff, Kathy Walsh, Barbra Johnston, Eileen Lukaszewski, Robert Thomson, and Deborah Liss Fins, provided invaluable editing expertise.

Rabbi Gary Klein, my spiritual teacher, whose insight, wisdom and many sermons have influenced my views on community, its essence and how I integrated this information into daily practice

I have been influenced by staff members (some of whom are deceased) at the hospitals in which I have worked: Morton Plant and Mease Hospitals: Drs. Wade Hatcher, Pete May, Don Eubanks, Mike Williamson, Paul Phillips, Joe Eaddy, Mark Michelman, Harry Wilks, Lee Watkins, Michael Andriola, Kerry Kaplan, Eric Weston,

Larry Zeitlin, and Al Schick. Watching their mannerisms and body language provided me with considerable insight and inspiration.

Ben Schaffer, who has been my office partner for the past decade and a half has been a sounding board for my ideas and a gentle guide along the way. Blair Holtey stands out as a guide and supporter in his position as hospital chaplain.

My medical office staff has been an invaluable source of encouragement and assistance. Vicki Pine became a great friend as an office manager for 18 year and has always been one of my biggest fans. Arlene Mitchell who succeeded Vicki and filled a set of shoes that I thought could ever be filled. Arlene's husband, Matt Mitchell has provided invaluable creation of my web and social media presence. And Mari Harper has been helpful as well in the area of social media.

I credit the many close friends and colleagues who listened to my tales and encouraged me to continue to endure through this painstaking process.

Book Club Questions and Topics for Discussion

1. What was unique about the structure of the book?
2. How did the structure enhance or take away from the book?
3. What specific themes did the author emphasize throughout the book?
4. What are these themes trying to get across to the reader?
5. Do the characters seem real and believable? Can you relate to their predicaments? To what extent do they remind you of yourself or someone you know?
6. In what ways do the events in the books reveal the author's view about aging?
7. Did certain parts of the book make you uncomfortable? If so, why did you feel that way?
8. Did these feelings lead to a new understanding or awareness of some aspect of life you might not have thought about before?
9. What did you find surprising about the facts introduced in this book?
10. How has reading this book changed your opinion of Aging GRACEfully??
11. How does the author present information in a way that is interesting and insightful?

12. If the author is writing on a debatable issue, does he give proper consideration to all sides the debate or does he appear to have a bias?

13. How has the book increased your interest in the subject matter?

14. Do the issues affect your life now or will they affect them in the future?

15. What type of language does the author use? Does this enhance the purpose of the book or deter from it? Explain.

16. What are the implications for the future in aging? How these implications do affects our lives now?

17. Does the author propose solutions? If so, who would implement those solutions and how probable is success?

18. How controversial are the issues raised in the book? Who is aligned on which sides of the issues? Where do you fall in that line-up?

19. What is the one point or idea that you have been left with after reading the book?

20. Pick one person from the book that you admired. One you detested. What life lesson can be learned from each?

21. Will you read other books by this author? Why or why not?

22. Did this book change your life in a positive or negative way? Explain

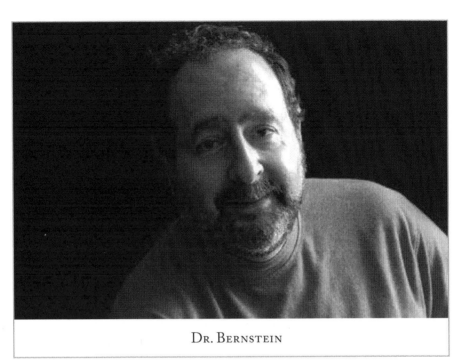

Dr. Bernstein

David Bernstein, MD is a highly respected physician who is board certified in both Internal Medicine and Geriatrics practicing in Clearwater, Florida. His 30 years of experience have provided him with opportunities to observe and empathize with thousands of adults as they age. His compassion and ability to see the souls of his patients has compelled him to share his stories in his book "I've Got Some Good News and Some Bad News: YOU'RE OLD Tales of a Geriatrician..."

He is a graduate of Albany Medical College and is an associate clinical professor in the department of medicine at the University Of South Florida College Of Medicine.

Dr. Bernstein is an avid public speaker, addressing various medical topics with his colleagues and with the community at large with a focus on families facing the complex problems as they near the end of life.

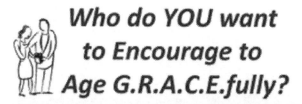

Who do YOU want to Encourage to Age G.R.A.C.E.fully?

Made in the USA
San Bernardino, CA
16 April 2016